MW01003073

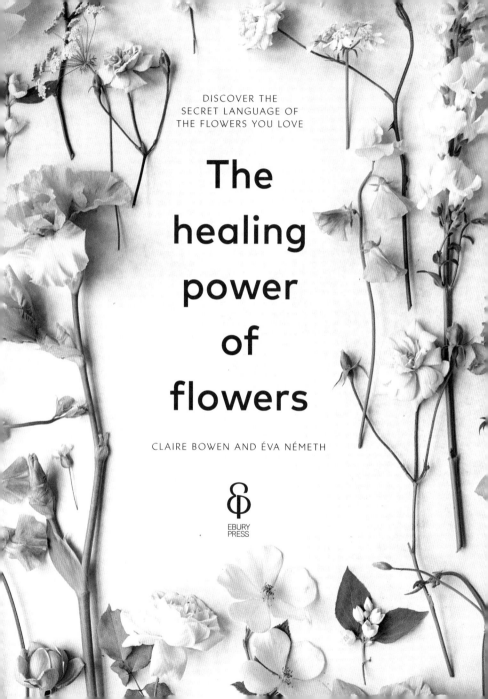

DISCOVER THE
SECRET LANGUAGE OF
THE FLOWERS YOU LOVE

The
healing
power
of
flowers

CLAIRE BOWEN AND ÉVA NÉMETH

EBURY
PRESS

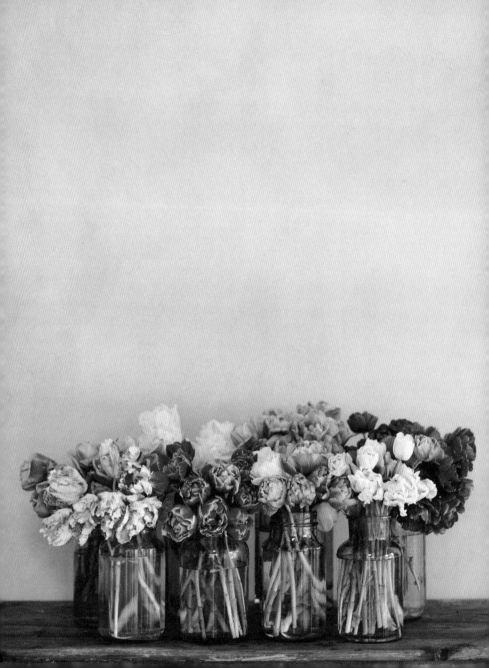

Introduction

Flowers are incredible. They have the power to calm, to heal and they allow us to express our deepest emotions without saying a word. They can boost your mood, reduce stress and improve well-being. By crafting thoughtful, personal bouquets, or choosing a flower for its traditional meaning, natural energy or holistic properties, you can bring the benefits of the natural world into your home or workplace, and into the lives of loved ones. Picking the ideal bloom for the moment can become an act of self-care and arranging a colourful bouquet can be a form of therapy.

The giving and receiving of flowers has a long tradition dating back to the Ancient Greeks, Romans and Egyptians. Flowers feature in Celtic myth and Druid beliefs. The Druids had many uses for plants, not just for eating and drinking but for medicinal purposes, in ritual ceremonies, as offerings and even to predict the future. Flowers have always enjoyed a privileged position in Chinese culture, too, not just in everyday life, but in art, literature and poetry, and many meanings for blooms originate from China.

Flowers take on symbolic meanings in legends, folklore and religious practices and play an important part in many customs and rituals across the globe. They continue to be a way for us to express complex emotions: to mourn, to comfort and to celebrate. They have maintained a prominent place in many cultures as a source of inspiration for both paintings and literature and are influential in many other forms of art – from furnishings and textiles to tattoos. As a florist, to be able to bring joy to a happy couple's wedding day with beautiful bouquets or a venue decorated with flowers, is a great privilege. Arranging a funeral spray or filling a chapel with a family member's favourite flowers upon their death is deeply cathartic, and in this sense, very little has changed since ancient times.

Modern life is complex. More and more of us find ourselves committed to busy routines, far removed from the natural world and its rhythmic cycles, and yet we are also becoming increasingly aware of the benefits that a little nature can bring. The idea that we already have enough and that our overconsumption contributes to widespread environmental problems is prevalent in people's minds and we want to know what we can do, in our own small way, to help protect the natural world while still being part of it. Crafting low-impact, natural gifts with real meaning is a wonderful place to start. By foregoing imported flowers with heavy carbon footprints and making floral choices based on the seasons, we can reduce our environmental impact, become more in tune with nature and celebrate the beauty that it has to offer.

As well as reducing carbon footprints, using locally grown flowers is one of the best ways to ensure the welfare of the growers. The global floral industry is not so different to other plant-based industries, like tea, coffee and cotton. Just as we seek out products that are Fairtrade, farmed by workers under safe conditions, or look for organic cotton that hasn't been sprayed with pesticides, so too should we seek the same from our flowers. Extra consideration for how your flowers are grown helps to ensure that you are supporting ethical businesses.

Expressing love and respect for flowers is a way to honour nature and helps you to tune in to the changing seasons and what they offer. This should influence the flowers that you choose; seasonal flowers grown locally are not only a more environmentally friendly option, they can also look very different from those that have been chemically treated and/or shipped in from overseas. Local flowers have a greater character and range – instead of poker-straight stems and stiff petals, you'll find a variety of shades and nuances of texture, crooked stems, wispy tendrils and fluffy, blousy blooms. They will be fresher, and so last longer, making them better value for money, too. Choosing seasonal flowers doesn't just help the planet, it will also improve your floral skills enormously. Learning to work with flowers that are in season will open up a world of blooms that you might not have considered before. Unusual varieties and colours, and twists and shapes will add extra dimensions to your bouquets and arrangements.

How to use this book

This book is a guide to help you learn more about the healing language of flowers.

When choosing your flowers there are many factors to consider. Do you want to go big and bold with a bouquet or small and whimsical with a single bloom? Decisions on colour, form and texture all play a part (see the section on How to make a simple bouquet, page 189). This book takes the message that you want the floral gift to send as the starting point, drawing upon the meanings and energies of the flowers. Each chapter addresses an emotional theme – celebration, joy, love, success, consolation and calm – and lists the flowers that suit this feeling, along with some explanation as to why. It includes suggestions for how to present them, instructions to make them into bouquets, plus tips on how to dry or press them to create lasting gifts.

As a book about floral language, the main questions is: 'If flowers can speak, what is it that we would like them to say?'. We want to use flowers to express messages of positivity and kindness. As well as drawing upon some of the more traditional meanings, the holistic properties of plants are also mentioned.

I've considered the natural energy that a flower imparts, too. In the past, some flowers have been attributed with negative meanings – hellebores, for instance, were supposed to represent lies and scandal and foxgloves were associated with falsehood. But the focus of this book is on healing, so I've sought the good in each and every flower, sometimes considering the role that it might play in the garden. Hellebores, which thrive in the coldest months and are long-lasting and durable, represent longevity and constancy, and foxgloves, standing tall and pretty in the flowerbed while bees buzz busily around them, are associated with productivity and success. These meanings differ from some that you might find in a more traditional book, but, while they are my own take on floral meanings, they use nature and outdoors as their point of reference.

Each entry lists the flowering period of that plant and when it is likely to be available, plus advice on how best to care for it. This is an approximate guide, as some may flower earlier or later, depending on whether it was a particularly mild winter or a very harsh one. Likewise, there will be regional variations and flowers may bloom on either side of the times listed here, depending on where you are in the world. The purpose of this guide is to help you plan what to seek out and check for availability, and also to help you realise that if you see peonies in February or roses in December, these will have been imported from much further afield, incurring a greater carbon footprint than flowers grown locally. Some of the flowers featured in this book are toxic when ingested and could pose a risk to households with inquisitive pets or small children. These flowers have been marked with a toxic symbol ⚠ so that you can choose your flowers with extra care.

How to care for your cut flowers

Once you have your flowers, remove any leaves on the stems that will end up beneath the water level in the vase. Fill your vase as high up to the top as you can without there being any danger of the water spilling over. Any leaves that remain below the water level will rot and feed bacteria, which will turn your water into an unpleasant swamp and will also prevent the stems from taking up water.

It is really important to keep your flower snips and any vessels that will hold the flowers scrupulously clean, as any dirt will have an adverse effect on the vase life of your blooms.

Trim your stems at a 45-degree angle before placing them in the water, cutting off the bottom few centimetres, depending on the original length of the stem.

To extend the vase life of your flowers if you are making a bouquet or arrangement, once you have removed the unwanted leaves it is a good idea to let the stems rest in water for 3–4 hours to properly hydrate. If you have unopened buds of flowers, such as roses, lilies or peonies, give them a drink of warm water to hurry them along gently.

Once you have made your bouquet or arrangement, trim another centimetre or two from the stems before putting them into water.

If you have bought a ready-made bouquet from a shop, or have received a bouquet from a friend, then trim the stems when you get home and place in water immediately.

Ensure that you trim the ends of your stems regularly, maybe every other day, and refresh the vase water daily. This is a much more effective, and environmentally friendly, option than using chemicals to extend the life of your flowers.

Keep your flowers in a cool spot, away from direct sunlight, for the longest vase life possible. Place them away from ripening fruit and vegetables which may emit ethylene, a gas that has no colour or odour and is often referred to as 'the ripening hormone'. Any flowers nearby are susceptible to absorbing this, which in turn leads them to ripen, or rather to die, more quickly.

Finally, remember that vase life varies dramatically from flower to flower – some are fleeting blooms, others long-lasting – this is part of their joy and unique charm. For the purpose of this book, it is fair to assume that most blooms will last for between three and five days, depending on factors like how long ago the flowers were picked before they were purchased (if buying from a florist or similar) and also the weather at the time – hot weather invariably leads to shorter vase life. Flowers that require specific care or are particularly short-lived or long-lasting are noted in their entry.

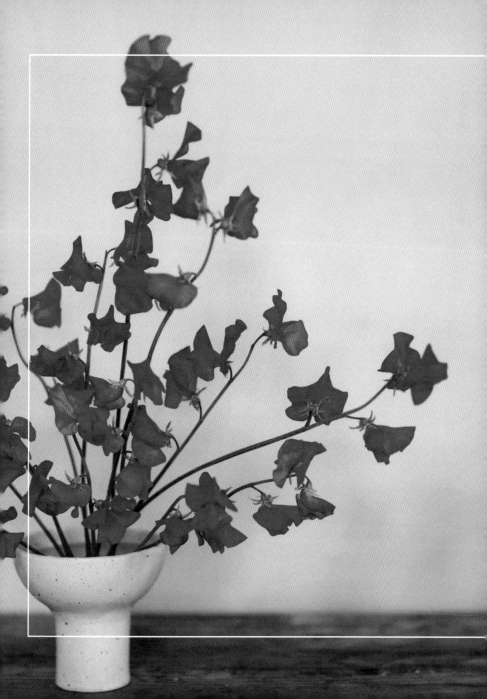

Flowers

for

<u>Joy</u>

Ranunculus

⊕ CARE The stems of cut
ranunculus can start to smell
very quickly if left untended.
However, if the ends are
trimmed regularly and their
water is changed daily, these
flowers should last for well
over a week. Their stems are
very fragile and snap easily,
so be careful when handling
them. If there are smaller
buds on the stems coming
off the main stem, try
trimming them off and
placing them in water – they
may well flower later and
you can observe the process
outlined above all over again.

⚭ PRESENTATION
A beautiful focal flower
as part of a bouquet or
arrangement, they are also
pretty in a jug or vase on
their own, either in one
colour or a variety.

⚠ TOXIC

Named after the Latin word for frog, *rana*, and
part of the buttercup family, these lollipop-shaped
flowers come in a variety of shades, ranging from
very dark reds and purples to candy-coloured
white, pale pink, bright pink, warm orange,
coral and yellow, reflecting the sweetness you
might find in a box of sugar mice.

When first cut, ranunculus are wrapped tightly
shut, revealing only the very outer layers. They
open slowly to expose their complex structure,
their layers gradually unfurling as if in very slow
motion. Very slow indeed, for this stage can take
up to a week. Once fully opened, they take on a
different shape entirely as their petals relax and
their colour is revealed, almost as if they have
burst open with happiness. The pink ones have
even been likened to little ballerinas in their
tutus, waiting in turn to pirouette across a stage.
Rather like the frogs from which they take their
name, they might even be jumping for joy!

Their uplifting energy and appearance mean
they are the perfect gift to bring joy to someone
when they need it most.

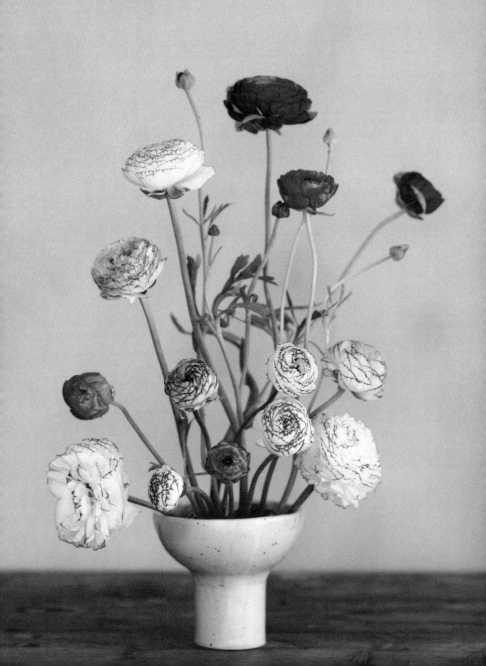

Cosmos

FLOWERING PERIOD
June to September

CARE Trim ends regularly
and refresh water daily.
Take care of these fragile
flowers as their petals
can bruise easily.

PRESENTATION
Perfect for adding a floaty
element to any bouquet or
arrangement, but add them
last to make sure they are
not crushed by bigger and
heavier flowers. They are
also lovely on their own in
a glass jar or vase.

With their yellow centres and white or pastel-coloured petals, these pretty blooms look much like the flowers we first think of when we conjure up childhood memories of summer. Similar in shape to a daisy, only bigger and a little more sophisticated, cosmos cannot fail to bring a smile to your face.

Their long stems are multi-headed, meaning there is more than one flower per stem, which makes cosmos good value, and they have delicate foliage which gives them a feeling of lightness. They are charming and happy flowers that make a great present for someone who needs a little joy in their life. They would also be perfect to celebrate a joyous occasion, such as the arrival of a new family member with their own childhood ahead of them.

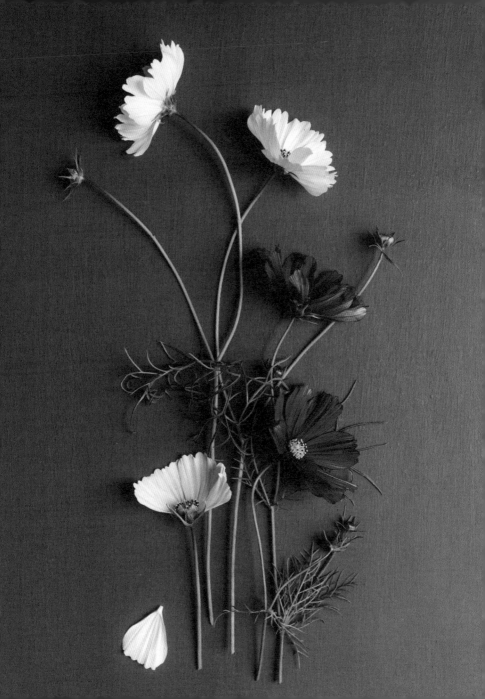

Spirea

⚜ **FLOWERING PERIOD**
April to May

⊕ **CARE** Crush, cut or break
woody branches in an
upwards motion, leaving
a larger cut surface area
so that more water can be
taken in. Trim the ends and
replace water daily to help
the blossom stay fresh as
long as possible. As the
branches get older, the
tiny petals will drop.

♣ **PRESENTATION**
Beautiful as a filler in
a bouquet, or on its own
in a vase with little or no
other adornment.

Frothy and light, spirea is in fact a deciduous
shrub that is part of the rose family, but it's
so pretty that it's often sold as a cut flower
at flower markets and in shops.

Coming into its own in spring, when it puffs
up into a glorious display of fluffy white flowers,
spirea gives off a joyful energy, signifying the
arrival of sunshine and fertility. It represents
renewal and the start of wonderful things
to come.

The sight of spirea growing outdoors is a beautiful
marker of spring and gathering some indoors,
or incorporating it into a floral piece, brings that
sense of lightness with it. It's the ideal token to
bring joy into someone's life and home.

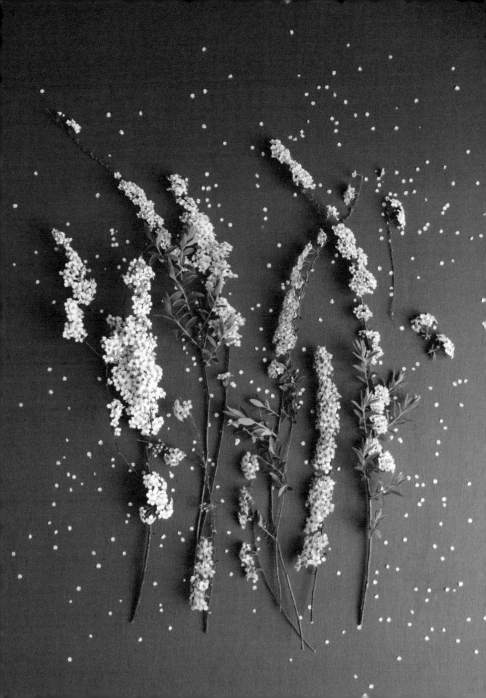

Ammi majus

⊛ FLOWERING PERIOD
May to August

⊕ CARE Trim the ends
regularly and refresh their
water daily and ammi will
last well over a week.

⚬ PRESENTATION
Ammi can grow more
than two metres tall, which
makes it perfect for large
arrangements. It can be
found in smaller lengths,
too, and with its floaty
structure it's ideal in
arrangements of all sizes
as well as bouquets. It is
also a good flower to dry.

With dainty white flowers grouped together
that resemble puffs of lace seemingly floating
above thin green stems, ammi is loved by florists
for its floaty, ethereal quality.

In the garden, ammi attracts butterflies and
other beneficial pollinator insects, and when
it has finished flowering, its seed heads provide
feed for the birds. It not only brings joy to the
eye but also to many garden inhabitants, and its
energy is positive and beneficial. It is easy to see
why ammi is traditionally an emblem of haven
and sanctuary, and it's a good present to give to
someone seeking a little joy in their life.

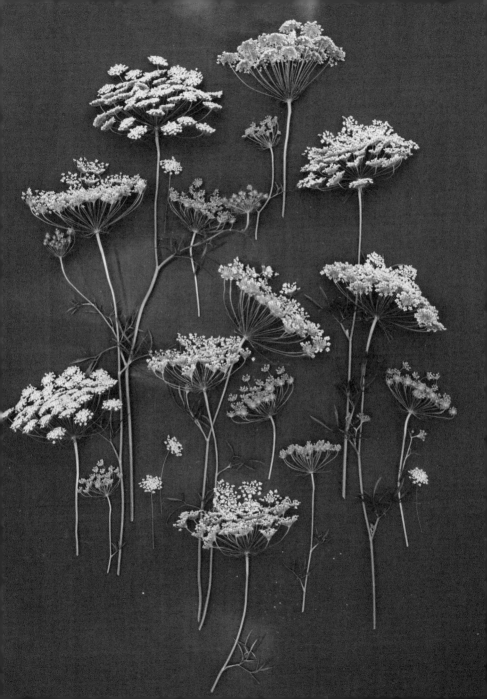

Delphiniums

FLOWERING PERIOD
May to August

CARE Trim stems regularly
and refresh water daily.
Delphiniums are very
sensitive to ethylene, so
keep them away from ripe
fruit. (see page 011).

PRESENTATION
Big bunches of these tall,
beautiful flowers look
great in large vases. They
are also particularly good
in arrangements where you
want some height. When
dried, the individual petals
make perfect confetti.

TOXIC

The delphinium gets its name from the Greek
word *delphus*, meaning 'dolphin', as the spur at
the top of the flower resembles a dolphin's head.
These stunning flowers have very long stems
covered in smaller flower heads and make a big
impact wherever they are used.

Delphiniums come in a variety of colours –
white, lilac, pale pink, pale blue, dark blue and
even deep purple. Blue, the most common colour,
represents dignity, while the white, pink and
light blue flowers are said to symbolise youth
and renewal. Whichever colour you choose, they
cannot fail to bring a smile to the recipient's face.

Just as its namesake the dolphin is associated
with playfulness and elation, the delphinium,
with its positive energy in the garden, waving
cheerfully at the back of the flowerbeds as bees
buzz in and out of its petals, is surely the
embodiment of joy in floral form.

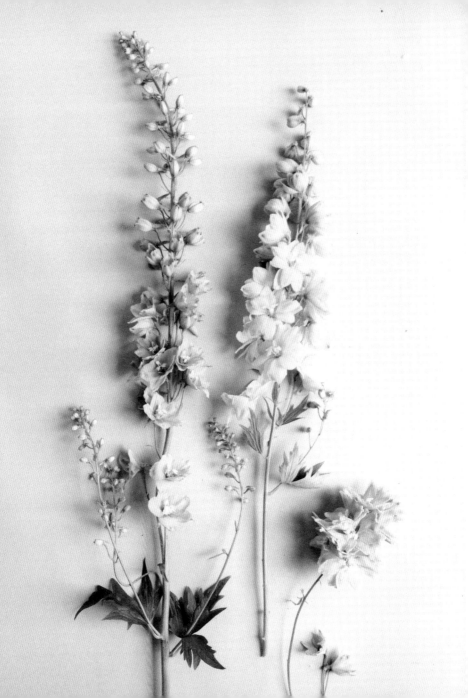

Buttercups

FLOWERING PERIOD
April to October

CARE Trim ends regularly and refresh water daily.

PRESENTATION
As these flowers are very small, with short stems, they are not appropriate for bouquets or arrangements, but look best bunched in a glass or small vase.

TOXIC

These tiny flowers are modest yet beautiful. For many they bring back memories of carefree, childhood summer days, so it's hardly surprising that they are emblems of cheerfulness and childhood. They are also said to represent charm and humility.

Although they are not the most luxurious of flowers, they still make a lovely gesture, and someone who appreciates simplicity will enjoy their humble beauty.

The buttercup's yellow colour symbolises optimism, new beginnings, joy and positivity, which makes them the perfect flower to cheer up someone's day.

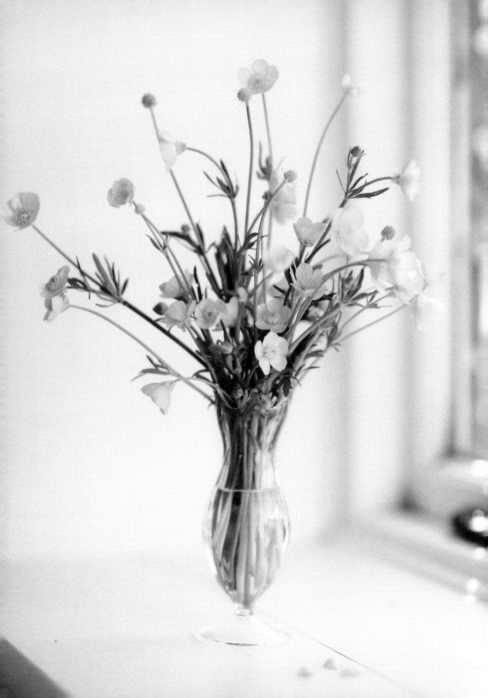

Sweet Peas

FLOWERING PERIOD
May to September

CARE Trim ends regularly
and refresh water daily
to get the maximum vase
life possible.

PRESENTATION As
sweet peas have relatively
short stems, they often
look prettiest when
arranged in small vases
by themselves, although
they also make good filler
flowers in both bouquets
and arrangements.

One of the most popular summer flowers, sweet peas are an all-time favourite. Their ruffled blooms and incredible scent make them one of the most charming and sought-after cut flowers.

The sweet pea's scientific name, *Lathyrus odoratus*, is derived from the Greek word *lathyros,* meaning 'pea', and the Latin word *odoratus,* meaning 'fragrant' – an apt description for this member of the pea family. There are many varieties of sweet pea and they are available in almost every colour except yellow.

It is perhaps because of their lovely smell and appearance that they are said to denote delicate or blissful pleasures, and a bunch of these have a joyful impact on all our senses.

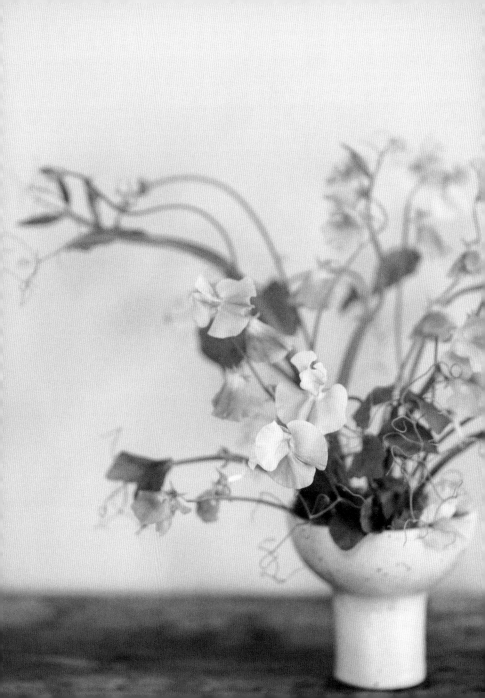

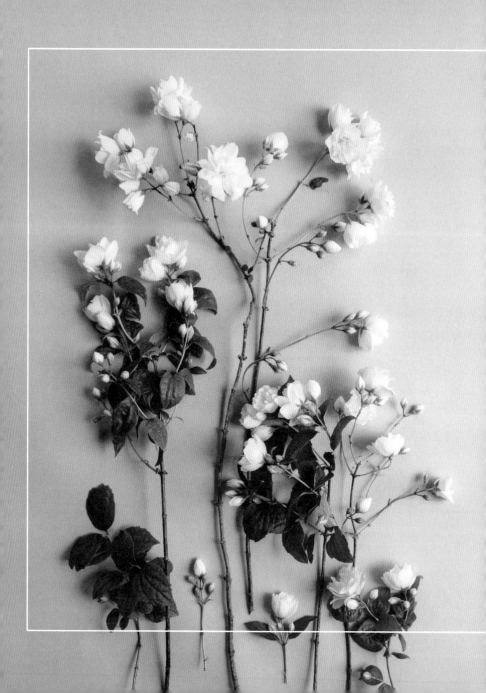

Flowers

for

<u>Calm</u>

Muscari

FLOWERING PERIOD
March to April

CARE Trim ends and refresh water daily to ensure longer vase life.

PRESENTATION Either give a small bunch of muscari on their own, or weave into a bouquet or arrangement.

These little flowers, commonly known as grape hyacinths because of their grape-like structure, are not to be confused with hyacinths, which are much larger (see page 160). They come into their own mid-spring when they carpet woodlands and shady gardens. You can increasingly find the bulbs being sold in florists and gift shops ready to be potted up into pretty vessels, or buy them as cut flowers to add a pop of blue to a room, arrangement or bouquet.

Muscari have a spicy, grape-like smell and their colour is bright and welcoming. Hues vary from dark violet and deep lapis blue to very pale blue and occasionally white, but it is the deep blue varieties that you see most often.

Traditionally, muscari stands for softness and caring love, while the colour symbolism for blue includes trust, loyalty, intelligence and faith but it is most strongly associated with tranquillity and calm.

Muscari would be an appropriate gift for someone in need of a little calm in their life but is also a good choice if you want to express loyalty.

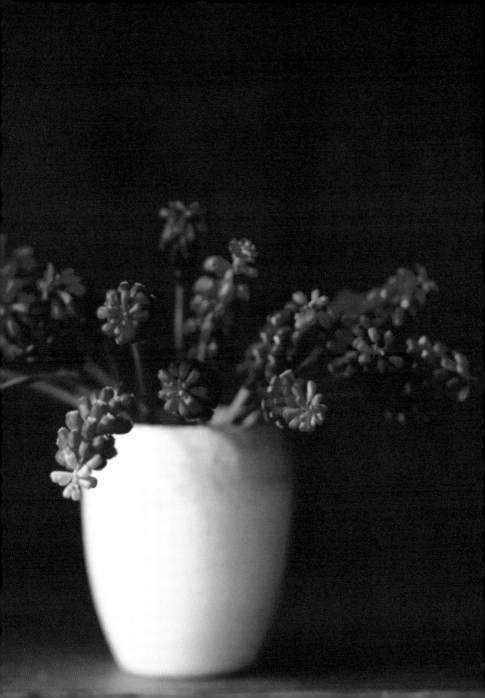

Jasmine

FLOWERING PERIOD
June to August

CARE Trim ends regularly
and refresh water daily. As
jasmine is twisty and curly,
it can move in the vessel
quite easily, so ensure that
stems are always below the
water level and don't slip
out. Once the flowers die
off, remove the blooms and
return the leaves, which will
still look nice, to the vase.

PRESENTATION Jasmine
adds a wonderful gestural
element to bouquets and
arrangements, but also
looks great in a big, tangled
bunch in a vase, or trailing
downwards in accordance
with its natural tendency.

Trailing jasmine is one of the most beautiful
floral sights as its long, dark grey shoots droop
over walls and doorways with a profusion of
silvery white flowers perfuming the air.

There are over 200 species of jasmine, many
of which originated in tropical and subtropical
areas. Forty-three different species of jasmine
are grown in East India, where it is known as
the King of Fragrance and the Moonlight of
the Grove. Its name comes from the Persian
word *Yasmin*, meaning 'gift from the gods'. It
is the national flower of Pakistan and is used in
religious ceremonies throughout Thailand and
the Philippines. Although it originates from
Asia, jasmine is now grown worldwide, and
many gardeners add it to their spaces.

Jasmine is used as an ingredient in many perfumes.
As well as smelling wonderful, it has very distinct
aromatherapeutic properties and is used to
soothe headaches, insomnia, grief, depression,
fear and worry. It is also said to boost energy.

With its cheerful disposition and distinctive
calming properties, jasmine makes a wonderful
present for someone seeking tranquillity and
rest. Its soothing aroma fills a home with a
sense of well-being.

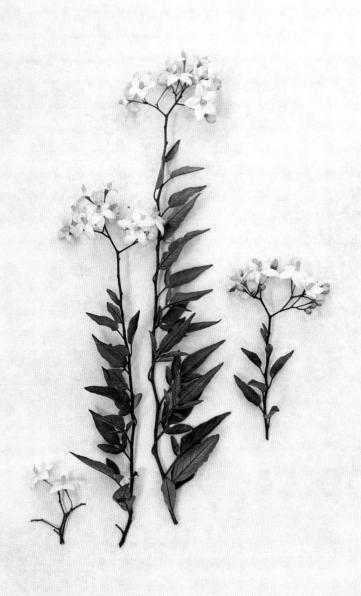

THE LANGUAGE OF

Quince

 FLOWERING PERIOD
March to May

CARE Trim woody stems
regularly and cut a 'V' shape
into them so that they can
soak up the maximum amount
of water. Refresh water daily.
Cared for correctly, these
flowers have a vase life of
at least a week.

PRESENTATION As
these beautiful flowers
come on quite straight,
twiggy branches, they look
best grouped together in
a jug, or as just one or two
stems in a vase. They can
be used as part of an
arrangement, but their
inflexible stems make them
less easy to work with than
some other flowers.

One of the very first flowers to appear on trees
at the end of winter, the coral hues of the quince
signal the approach of spring and the end of long,
dark nights. Originally from Asia and very popular
in Japanese imagery, quince are now grown
across the world and admired for their delicate
buds and great beauty as well as their fruit.

In natural medicine, quince is anti-inflammatory
and used as a soothing astringent to treat coughs
– in Japan quince cough sweets are commonly
sold in pharmacies – and applied to burns.
Its job in nature is to calm and to heal.

Quince's remedial properties make it the perfect
gift for someone in need of calm, perhaps when
recovering from an illness, in need of rest, or
coming out of a turbulent time and seeking
some comfort and reassurance.

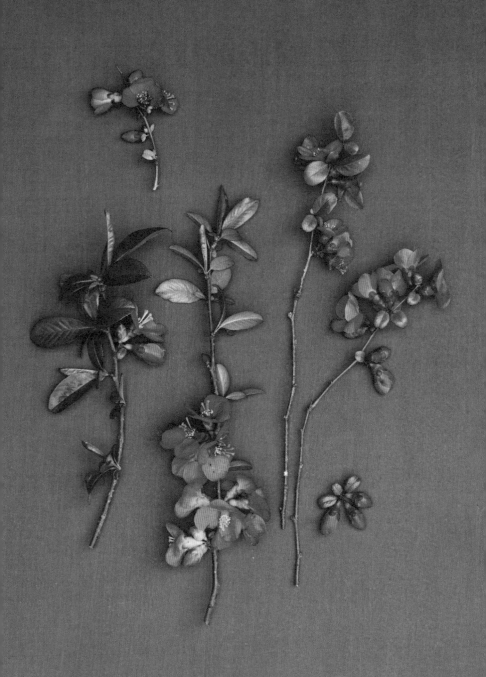

Japanese Anemones

⚜ FLOWERING PERIOD
July to October

⊕ CARE Trim ends regularly
and refresh water daily.

⚱ PRESENTATION
Japanese anemones have
a wonderfully floaty nature
and are ideal in both bouquets
and mixed arrangements.

⚠ TOXIC

Sometimes confused with the brightly coloured anemones that flower in spring, Japanese anemones bloom from late summer through to the first frost. These delicate flowers range from white to pale pink in colour and are sometimes referred to as windflowers.

Despite their name, these anemones actually originate in China, but the Japanese later claimed them for their own as they became a feature of their iconic ornamental gardens.

Japanese ornamental gardens are created to inspire peace and contemplation and these flowers were introduced to contribute to the overall feeling of calm and serenity. They're an ideal token to give to someone wanting a little peace and tranquillity in their own life.

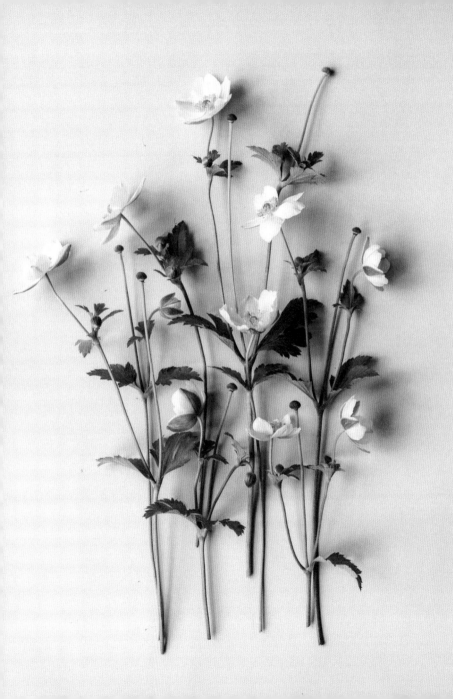

Solomon's Seal

FLOWERING PERIOD
May to June

CARE Trim ends regularly
and refresh water daily.

PRESENTATION These
elegant stems sit well in
bouquets, giving them some
structural shape, and also
look good in arrangements.

TOXIC

Solomon's seal has a lovely long stalk with
alternating deep green leaves that produce little
white flowers which dangle prettily underneath.
The seals in the base of the plant where the stalks
rise up from the ground are said to resemble
sigils, symbols used by magicians (usually
circles with symbols inside them). The word
'sigil' itself derives from the Latin *sigillum*,
meaning 'seal'. The plant is strongly associated
with magical properties and was named after
the wise King Solomon.

Solomon's seal has many healing properties
and herbalists use it to support and strengthen
the body by soothing inflamed tissue and to ease
chest and throat infections. It is also said to have a
mild sedative effect, soothing nervousness, distress
and irritation. Solomon's seal tea is sold to aid
a range of ailments from inflammation after
exercise to gastrointestinal inflammation. It has
been used in Asia for many centuries in different
forms, from herbal tinctures or salves to a
supplement in a pill.

This beautiful and elegant plant makes an
excellent gift for someone in search of a calm
and soothing influence.

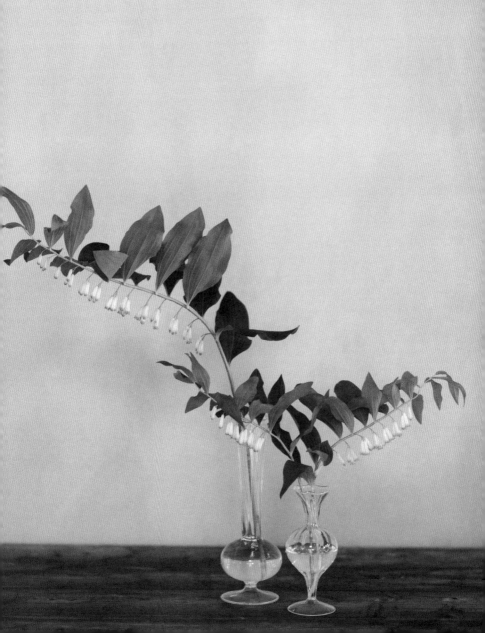

Mock Orange

FLOWERING PERIOD
May to June

CARE Trim woody stems
regularly and refresh
water daily.

PRESENTATION
These wonderful flowers
are attached to elegantly
curved, small branches,
which make a particularly
good addition to any
bouquet. They also sit
well in arrangements,
adding some space and
light among the heavier
flowers, or can be put simply
in a vase or jug to shine on
their own.

Pretty white flowers grow on arching stems that hang from the mock orange *(Philadelphus)* tree. The name mock orange comes from the fact that at first the white blooms and the scent mirror that of an orange tree. For this reason, mock orange was traditionally said to have negative connotations of fraudulence and deceit.

There is no denying, however, that these fragrant white flowers, which have a scent similar to both orange and jasmine, are a worthy addition to any home, even if they aren't citrus blossoms. As well as their beauty, which can be further highlighted by paring back some of the leaves from the branches to focus on the delicate flowers, the fragrance of both orange and jasmine are known to have calming and relaxing properties in the world of aromatherapy, making mock orange a perfect gift for someone seeking tranquillity.

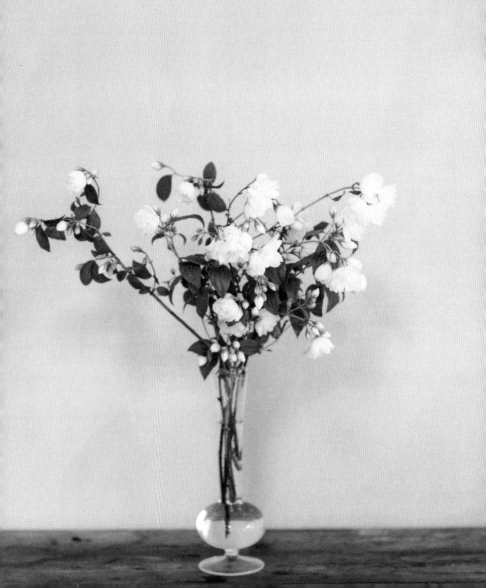

Verbena

FLOWERING PERIOD
June to September

CARE Trim ends regularly
and refresh water daily.

PRESENTATION Verbena
sits well in bouquets and
arrangements and adds a
floaty element to both.

Verbena, also commonly known as vervain, has purple-hued foliage and long slender stems topped with little spikes of flowers. In Ancient Rome, the herb was considered sacred and was placed on the altars in temples, while bunches of verbena twigs were used to sweep the temple. In the Middle Ages, it was thought that carrying verbena brought good luck, and it was also believed that if you rubbed verbena on your skin, then your wishes would be granted.

This latter belief is closest to the uses of verbena today. As well as making an attractive cut flower, verbena is used frequently in holistic medicine. Taken as a tea or tincture, it is believed to ease the nervous system, help relieve depression and is also used to reduce the symptoms of cold and flu. Applied directly to the skin, it is thought to aid arthritis. However you take it, and for whichever of these ailments, the overall effect of verbena is a calming one. Some sprigs of verbena are the perfect token to give to someone who needs a little soothing or a sense of tranquillity in their life.

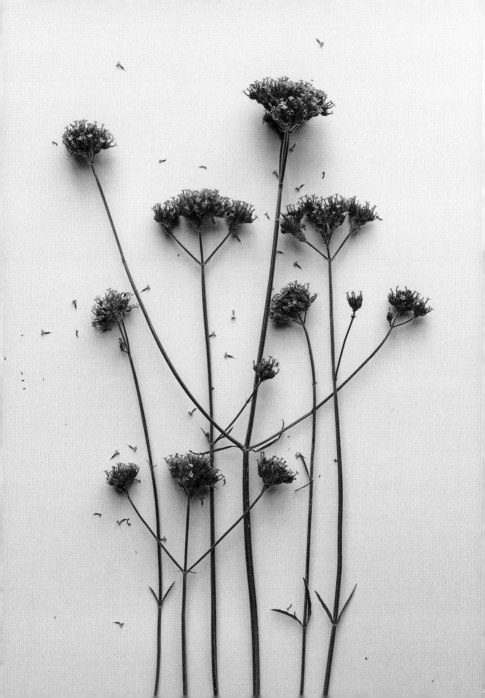

Snapdragons

FLOWERING PERIOD
June to September

CARE Trim ends regularly and refresh water daily.

PRESENTATION
Snapdragons look wonderful in both bouquets and arrangements alike. They also look good bunched in a glass vase or a jar.

The name snapdragon comes from the fact that if you squeeze the flower by its side it resembles a dragon's head. Its scientific name, *Antirrhinum*, comes from the Greek *anti*, meaning 'like', and *rhin*, meaning 'nose', which certainly seems like a good name for this snout-like plant.

Known to grow in rocky areas, the snapdragon's tenacity and ability to bloom in poor conditions has led to it being seen as a symbol of strength in trying circumstances. It is also said to represent graciousness. It is the perfect gift for someone who needs to be gracious under pressure and draw on their inner strength to help them appear calm and unflappable to the outside world.

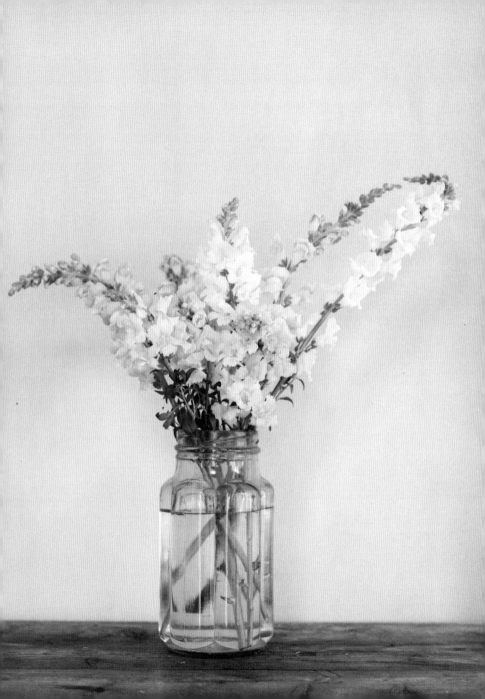

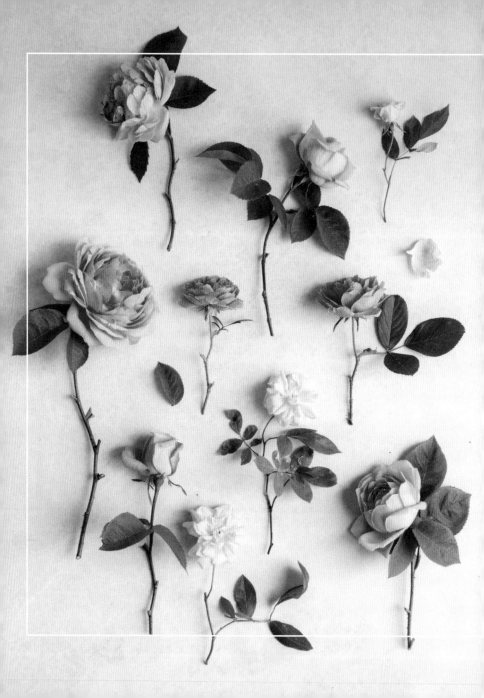

Flowers

for

<u>Love</u>

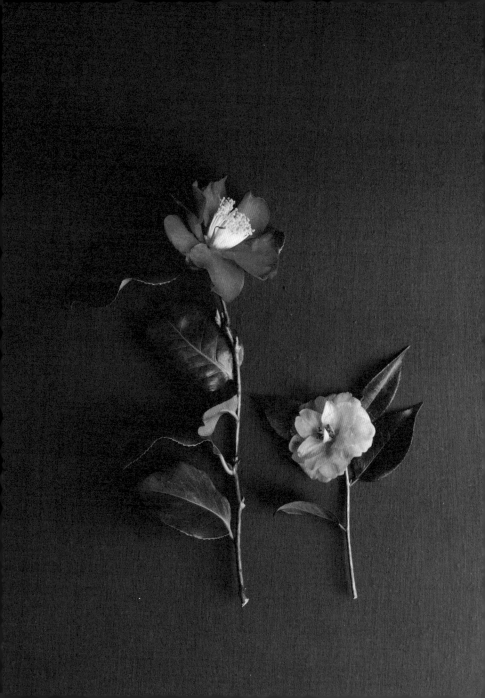

Camellias

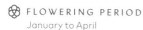 **FLOWERING PERIOD**
January to April

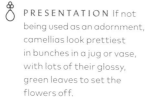 **CARE** If used as a
hairpiece or corsage and
out of water, their lifespan
is very short indeed, perhaps
just a few hours, but if kept
in water, camellias do well
as long as the ends are
regularly trimmed, and
the water is replaced daily.

PRESENTATION If not
being used as an adornment,
camellias look prettiest
in bunches in a jug or vase,
with lots of their glossy,
green leaves to set the
flowers off.

Perhaps most famous in modern times for
their association with the great fashion designer
Coco Chanel, for whom they were a timeless
symbol of elegance, these flowers, part of an
evergreen bush, are especially revered in Japan
where they grow wild. The camellia, or *tsubaki*,
as it is known in Japan, has always been
significant in Japanese culture. It is used as
a design motif for *noh* (theatre costumes) and is
prized in ikebana arrangements. Just as Japanese
cherry blossom is celebrated for its showiness,
the camellia is revered for the serene and quiet
beauty of its flowers and leaves.

The flower was named after Georg Kamel, who
brought the camellia to Europe from East Asia in
the eighteenth century. Camellias soon became
sought after as a luxury and Victorian ladies often
attended fancy dress balls either clutching a posy
of them, wearing them in their hair or even
dressed as a camellia!

Known as the Empress of Winter because they
bloom during late winter, as with many plants
the meaning varies according to the colour of the
flower: white represents perfect loveliness, pink
signifies longing and red tells the recipient that
they set the giver's heart on fire.

Phlox

⊛ FLOWERING PERIOD
June to September

⊕ CARE Phlox lasts
particularly well, sometimes
more than a week, if properly
cared for. Trim ends regularly
and refresh water daily.

⊗ PRESENTATION This
delicate, floaty flower looks
wonderful in both bouquets
and arrangements.

These pretty flowers come in a variety of
shapes and colours, mainly whites, pinks and
purples. They are especially popular in Japan,
where the Fuji Shibazakura Festival draws
large crowds to see up to 800,000 *shibazakura*,
which translates as 'lawn cherry' or 'pink moss',
so-called because of the way phlox completely
carpets the ground.

On a practical level, phlox is a reliable cut
flower that lasts well. In terms of symbolism,
it represents united souls, united hearts and long
friendships or is indicative of a reliable partner.
Phlox means unity and by giving it to someone
you can be sure you are sending a clear message
– if you have been feeling romantic and are
thinking about proposing to your loved one,
this is the flower with which to communicate
your feelings.

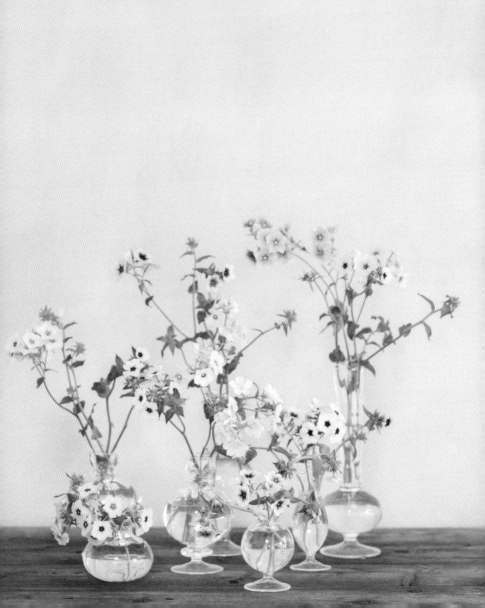

Nigella

CARE Trim ends regularly
and refresh water daily. The
stems are easily broken, so
handle with care.

PRESENTATION
Nigella looks great in both
bouquets and arrangements
and also on its own in a glass
vase or jar. You can leave
the wispy fronds on the
stems to add frothiness to
an arrangement or remove
them to attract attention
to the flower itself. It is
pretty either way.

Nigella is also known as love-in-the-mist because
of the fronds – the 'mist' – which look a little like
fennel and surround the delicate flower – the
'love'. This unassuming flower comes in shades
of pink, blue and white and, while pretty on its
own, it makes a very useful filler or floaty bloom
when nestled in between other flowers.

Given its alternative name, it would be difficult not
to associate nigella with love, but it is specifically
an emblem of delicacy and embarrassment as
well as love – in fact, it would be the ideal flower
to give to someone you are a little shy of revealing
your true feelings to.

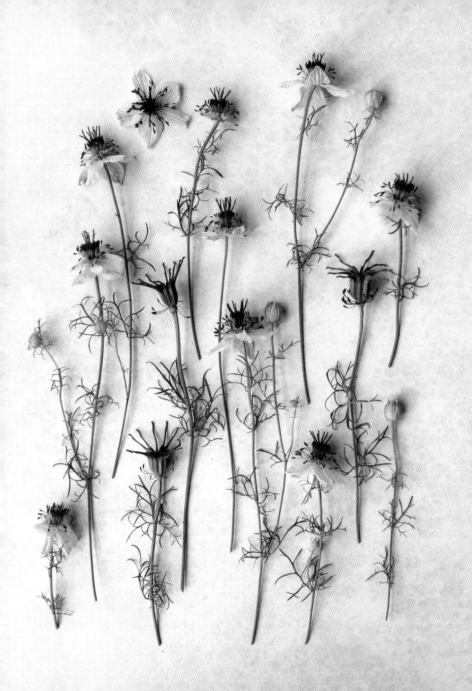

Carnations

FLOWERING PERIOD
June to September

CARE Trim ends regularly
and refresh water daily.
Carnations have a good
vase life if properly cared
for and can last for as
long as ten days.

PRESENTATION Pretty
as a bunch in a glass vase
or jar, carnations also sit
well in both bouquets and
arrangements.

Carnations have long been associated
with love, and with marriage in particular.
Renaissance paintings from the fifteenth and
sixteenth centuries by artists such as Albrecht
Dürer, Leonardo da Vinci and Raphael show
marriage partners holding a carnation as a
symbol of betrothal.

Different colours of carnation have various
meanings within the overall theme of love: pink
carnations are symbolic of pure and romantic
love; red ones signify ardent love and white tell
the recipient that they are fair and beautiful. With
their beauty and strong historical associations
with romance, carnations make the perfect gift
for the one you love.

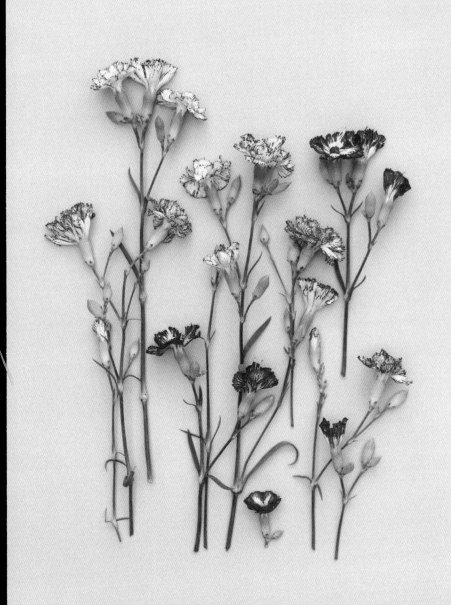

Bleeding Hearts

❀ **FLOWERING PERIOD**
April to May

⊕ **CARE** Trim stems and
replace water daily to
ensure flowers last as long
as possible. Properly cared
for, these cut flowers last
longer than most.

⚘ **PRESENTATION**
Beautiful as bunches in one
small vase, or dotted together
in several small vases,
these flowers also add airy
accents to arrangements
and bouquets.

This beautiful spring plant has heart-shaped blossoms dangling from arching stems which make charming cut flowers, and it is almost impossible not to associate it with love. Bleeding heart's name comes from its heart-shaped petals, which have a longer part at the bottom that resembles a tear, or a drop of blood, dripping from the petal. It is often said to symbolise rejected or unrequited love, especially in Eastern cultures. The flower has been cultivated for many centuries in Korea, China and Japan. Some have added further layers of meaning to include unconditional and compassionate love, the love of someone who loves the other no matter what. Certainly, it represents passion and sensitivity.

White bleeding hearts symbolise innocence and purity and are a wonderful gift for someone who is kind and generous. You can give this flower to a family member or friend who has supported and been there for you no matter what, or to someone who you will always be there for. Pink varieties, meanwhile, represent romance and love. They are the perfect present for your partner or the person you love, although you could also give them to a family member or a dear friend as a message of affection.

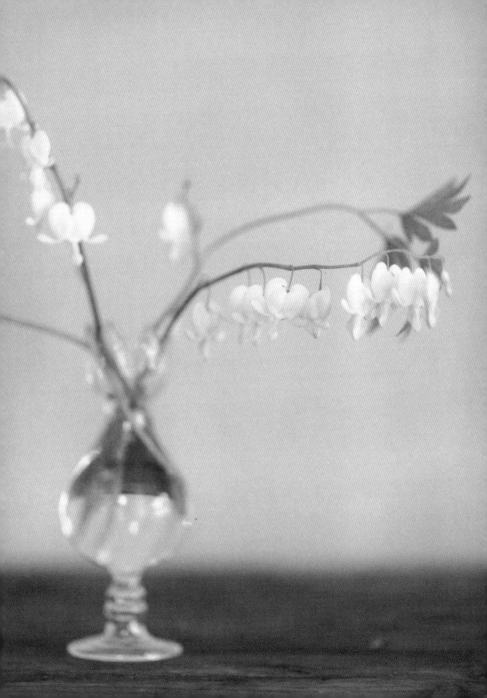

Bluebells

FLOWERING PERIOD
May

CARE Keep stems
trimmed regularly and
refresh water daily.

PRESENTATION As
these are small, delicate
flowers, they sit well as a
little bunch in a simple vase
or jar, but also look good
in small arrangements.

TOXIC

*The flower pictured here
is the Spanish variety.*

Bluebells are native to western Europe and many
thousands can grow in one woodland, creating
the incredible carpets of flowers that are one
of the joys of spring. As well as the familiar blue,
these little flowers can be found in shades of pink,
lilac and white. In addition to English bluebells,
which form a drooping 'C' shape with their
heads, there are Spanish bluebells, which are
distinguishable by their slimmer stem and upright
shape. A small bunch of bluebells, is a wonderful
way to bring the feeling of the outdoors inside, but
be aware it is illegal to pick them in the wild.

The bluebell is a symbol of gratitude, humility,
constancy and everlasting love. There are countless
folklores, tales and myths surrounding bluebells,
some of which involve fairy magic. Bluebells
are most often found in (ancient) woodlands
which are believed to be intricately woven
with fairy enchantments. It is said that if you
turn a bluebell flower inside-out without tearing
it, you will win the heart of the one you love, and
if you wear a wreath of bluebells you will only
be able to speak the truth. Bluebells have often
been included in traditional bridal bouquets
for this reason. A posy of these unmistakable
bell-shaped flowers is the perfect expression of
long-term love or constant friendship.

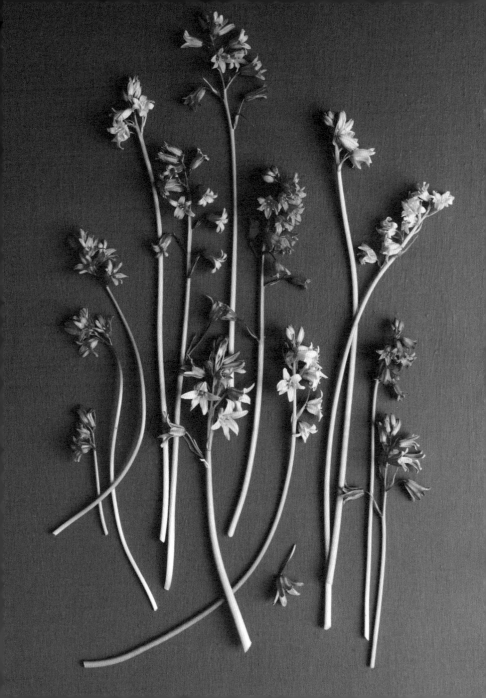

Forget-me-nots

FLOWERING PERIOD
April to June

CARE Keep stems trimmed and change water daily.

PRESENTATION
Forget-me-nots look lovely bunched together in a small glass vase or jar but can also be added to the front of bouquets and arrangements to add a 'pop' of blue.

The name of this flower clearly expresses its meaning, speaking of loyalty and lasting love (or friendship). It derives its name from a German folktale about two lovers who were walking on the banks of the Danube the day before their wedding. The bride-to-be admired some small, beautiful blue flowers and her fiancé stooped to pick them for her. He fell into the river and as he was swept away by the waters, he threw a bunch of the flowers at her feet, exclaiming, *'Vergiss mein nicht!'* ('Forget me not!').

Since then the flower has been used as a symbol of love and constancy, incorporated into Valentine's bouquets, painted onto china or embroidered onto fabric. If a soldier was going away to war, a locket with a forget-me-not engraved on it, containing a lock of the departed's hair, served as a reminder to his love of his constancy. This is the perfect flower to express love and faithfulness.

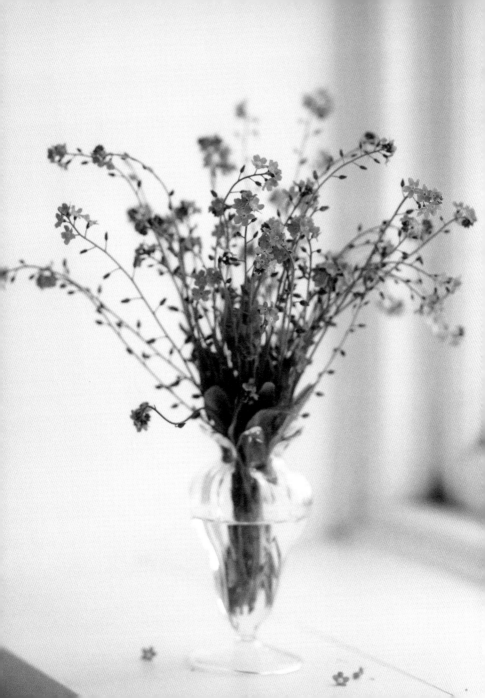

Honeysuckle

FLOWERING PERIOD
May to October

CARE Trim ends regularly and refresh water daily. As honeysuckle is twisty and curly, it can move in the vase quite easily, so ensure that stems are always below the water level and don't slip out.

PRESENTATION
Honeysuckle adds a wonderful gestural element to bouquets and arrangements, but also looks great in a big, tangled bunch in a vase.

TOXIC

Honeysuckle is a beautiful, cheerful climbing plant with a wonderful fragrance that has nothing but happy connotations. It is the symbol of devoted love, fidelity and loyalty. It is often seen climbing around the walls and doorframes of houses, clinging affectionately to trees, lattices and porches as it encompasses a home. It is no surprise that this sweet-scented flower, which gently hugs a house, is also the symbol of a contented home.

With all its connotations of long-lasting love and homeliness, honeysuckle is the perfect gift to give a loved one or partner, either as a gesture of long-established love, or as you enter into a new life together. It is an ideal gesture when moving into a new home together, or as a house-warming present for others.

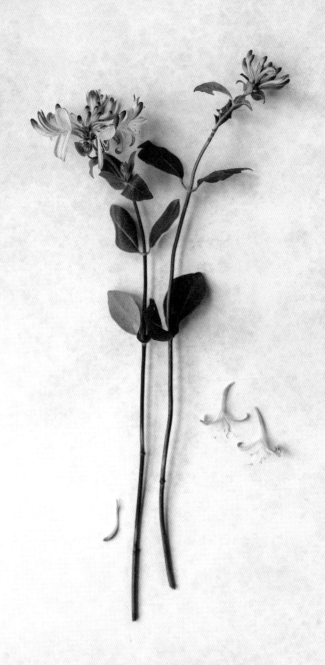

Campanula

FLOWERING PERIOD
June to September

CARE Trim ends regularly
and refresh water daily.

PRESENTATION This
little flower looks good
towards the bottom of an
arrangement or on its own
in a glass jar or vase.

This small plant, with its distinctive bell-shaped flowers dangling from its stems, is also known as the bell flower because the Latin word *campanula* means 'little bell'.

The campanula is an emblem of love and is associated with a myth that ties its origins to Venus, the Roman goddess of love. In Roman mythology, Venus had a mirror with magical powers whereby anyone who looked into it appeared to be beautiful. One day it was found by a young shepherd. Finding himself overwhelmed by happiness whenever he looked into it, he decided to keep it. Venus enlisted Cupid to help her find her beloved mirror. Cupid begged the shepherd to return the mirror, but he was already under its spell and refused to give it up. So, Cupid shot the shepherd's hand with an arrow to make him drop the mirror and as it hit the ground it shattered into many pieces – wherever a fragment fell, a campanula began to grow.

As well as its strong connections with love, the campanula is more specifically seen as a symbol of constancy and everlasting love. It is sometimes placed on graves for this reason. It's the perfect romantic flower to give to someone you treasure or even someone you like.

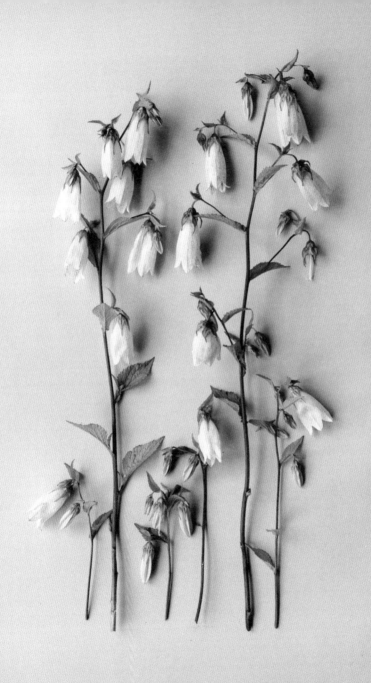

Clematis

⊛ **FLOWERING PERIOD**
May to July

⊕ **CARE** Trim ends regularly
and refresh water daily.

⬡ **PRESENTATION**
Clematis adds a light touch
to bouquets as the flowers
are at the top of the stem,
leaving the foliage further
down the stem to add some
greenery to your piece. It is
useful in arrangements for
the same reason, but also
looks pretty in a vase on
its own.

⚠ **TOXIC**

The Greek name *clematis* was originally used to describe a whole variety of climbing plants but is now used especially for this pretty climber, which is part of the buttercup family. Clematis is traditionally associated with love, emotional integrity and soulmates. When growing in the garden, like many climbing parts, this flower seems to be reaching for the sky, so it is not surprising that it should be associated with such lofty ideals, and its prettiness lends itself to the meanings of love and beauty.

This flower makes the perfect token to give to someone you love and admire for their inner beauty as well as their outward appearance, someone you want to be a constant part of your life.

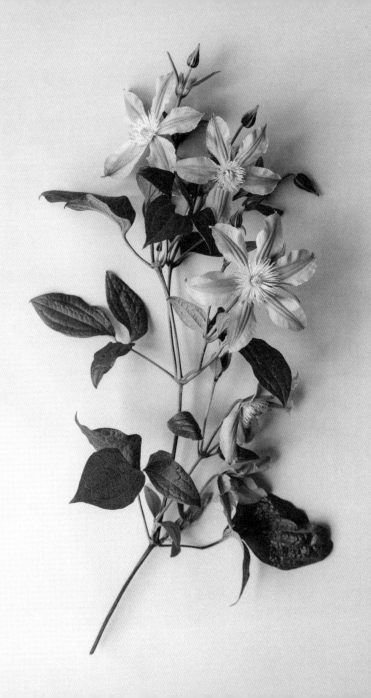

Dahlias

FLOWERING PERIOD
July to October

CARE Most dahlias only
last a few days. To keep
them for as long as possible,
pick off the petals at the
back as they begin to die.
Trim ends regularly and
refresh water daily.

PRESENTATION
These wonderful flowers
make a bold statement in
any bouquet or arrangement
but remember that their
lifespan is short. A mixture
of dahlia varieties in a vase
also looks very pretty.

The attention-seeker of the flower world, dahlias
come in many forms – spiky, cactus-shaped
flowers, pom-pom blooms and water-lily-shaped
varieties. They put on a bold and colourful display
in shades of pink, red, orange, yellow, brown,
white and dark burgundy. Almost every colour
except blue, in fact.

The dahlia is a flower that likes to make
an entrance, like a celebrity on the red carpet
or a model on the catwalk, and is traditionally
associated with dignity, good taste, refinement
and elegance as well as love. To the Victorians
in particular, the dahlia signified a strong
commitment to the person they were giving
it to. They would give dahlias to their partners
as a sign of their eternal love and to keep their
love alight. In keeping with its associations
with stylishness, Victorian ladies who considered
themselves at the height of fashion might plant a
dahlia walk (if their gardens were large enough!).
A grassy path would have borders of mixed
dahlias on either side and people could walk
in between admiring the blooms.

Dahlias make the perfect gift for someone you
love, especially someone with a strong sense of
style to whom this flower will appeal.

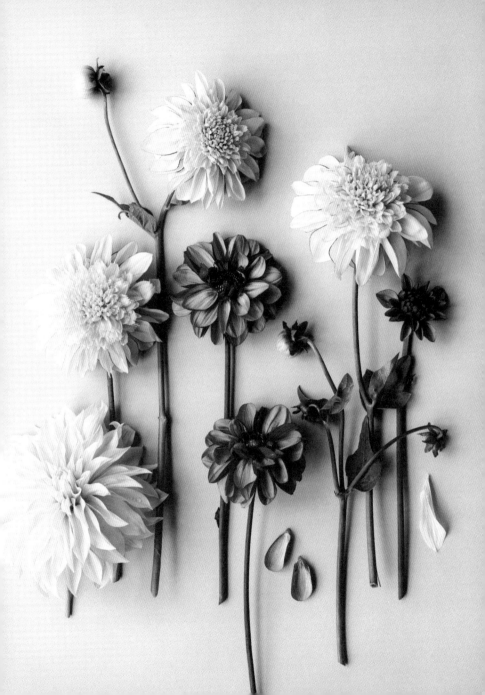

Lilies

FLOWERING PERIOD
June to July

CARE Lilies have pollen inside them that can stain clothes and fabric, so cut the stamens out of the centre before arranging the blooms. Trim ends regularly and refresh water daily and these flowers should last well.

PRESENTATION Lilies are such splendid flowers, with lovely long stems, that they look wonderful on their own in a tall vase. However, they can also be used as focal flowers within arrangements, or bouquets, assuming that the stamens have been removed.

TOXIC

Lilies, with their great beauty and tall and slender stems, have traditionally been revered for their majesty and grace. Although they have become less popular in recent years, perhaps due to their association with funerals, these scented blooms make a wonderful display in any home.

Lilies come in a variety of shades and colours, and each one has a slightly different meaning: pink ones signify prosperity, red are for passion, while yellow flowers represent thankfulness. It is the white lily, however, which symbolises purity and virtue, that we are most concerned with here.

Of all the lilies, it is the white Madonna lily that is the most sought after. The story of the Apostles opening the tomb of the Virgin Mary three days after her burial, and finding it empty with only roses and lilies in her place, led to many images of her holding, or being close to, a lily. For this reason, it is said to represent perfection of the highest order. Historically, perfect womanhood was represented by the Virgin Mary, and thus to compare a lady with a lily, or to give her this flower, was a very great compliment indeed.

Thus the lily, representing beauty, devotion and purity of heart has become a symbol of perfect love.

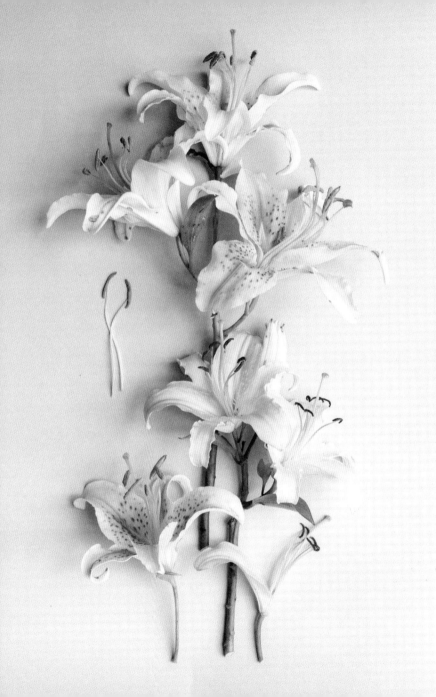

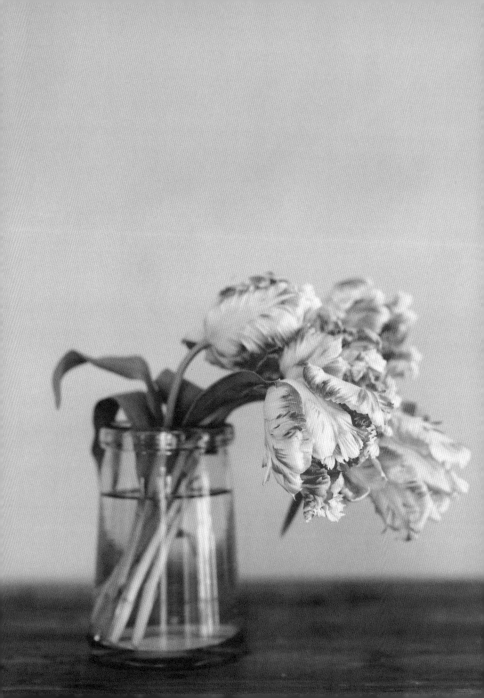

Tulips

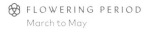

FLOWERING PERIOD
March to May

CARE If tulips appear floppy just after you have bought (or cut) them, wrap them in paper for support and place upright in a vase while they rehydrate. Tulips become increasingly beautiful as they age and their heads open up to reveal stunning petals; many will change colour and their stems will start to twist and curl, which only adds to their charm, so don't be too quick to discard them. Keep stems trimmed regularly and refresh water daily.

PRESENTATION With their heavy heads, tulips are good to use in arrangements, but they do better when they are supported by other nearby flowers. Alternatively, they look good in bouquets, or a simple bunch of tulips in a vase brightens up any room.

Such is our love of tulips that we even have a special expression for it – tulip mania.

The term was originally used to refer to an obsession with tulips that sprang up in Holland in the seventeenth century. Although tulips originated in the Middle East and were highly prized by the Turks, it was a seventeenth-century traveller, John Chardin, who introduced them to the Netherlands.

The mania that followed meant that people were sometimes prepared to pay huge sums of money – equivalent to the cost of a house – to obtain tulip bulbs. Bulb prices reached incredible heights and for a while were only within reach of the very richest members of society, but as their availability grew, so prices came down, and by the nineteenth century tulips had become more affordable for ordinary gardeners and flower lovers. The tulip was a flower that could in itself elicit huge amounts of love, infatuation even, and to give something so precious to another person was to imply true love indeed.

Different colours have subtle variations of meaning: strong, bright reds suggest a suitor is on fire with ardour, while striped tulips were traditionally used to mean 'you have pretty eyes' and yellow was seen as a sign of hopeless love. More recently, paler colours have also become popular and these shades reflect a softer, more romantic love, or can even be used as a gesture of friendship.

Just as the dramatic history of the tulip came about because of our passion for the flower, so it too is seen as a symbol of passionate love. Its purpose is to express love as much as it is to be loved itself.

Roses

⊕ CARE To get the maximum vase life from roses, submerge their stems in water and recut. If buying for special events, make sure that roses have time to rest and drink up water before you arrange them, anything from 24–48 hours. Warm water will encourage rosebuds to open. Trim ends regularly and refresh water daily thereafter.

⚲ PRESENTATION Roses are highly adaptable flowers, and as well as appearing in bouquets and arrangements, they are often used in buttonholes, flower crowns, and even as dried petals for confetti.

The rose is surely the perfect floral embodiment of love. There are literally thousands of varieties, from soft, old English roses, spray roses with smaller heads on multiple branches, and more structured roses such as tea roses, and many colours, too. The classic red rose says 'I love you' and represents passionate love, while white ones symbolise purity and innocence and are a popular choice for wedding flowers. Peach flowers represent modesty and sincerity and yellow roses, which the Victorians associated with jealousy, also convey wealth, cheer and general gladness. A mixture of red and white roses is said to represent unity. The number of roses can sometimes carry significance, too, be it a single rose, two roses to signify love and mutual affection, or three roses as a traditional one-month anniversary gift. A dozen roses is meant to be the ultimate romantic gesture, especially popular on Valentine's Day, but it is worth remembering that roses are not in season then, so these will have been flown in from overseas.

With huge popularity, there comes great demand, and unfortunately roses are one of the flowers most often imported, incurring significant carbon footprints. It is far, far better to choose local varieties and show love to the growers and the planet as well as to your beloved. (If you must buy roses out of season, check that they are Fairtrade.)

Luckily, increasing numbers of growers are selling their roses either directly or to local florists. These flowers will not only look more natural but will have a delicious scent that no manufactured rose ever could, and the fragrance that they give off is every bit as enticing as their appearance.

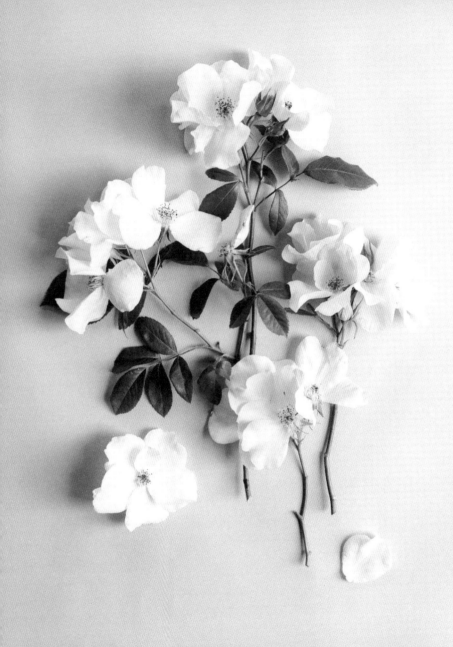

Lilacs

⊕ **FLOWERING PERIOD**
April to May

⊕ **CARE** As well as trimming the ends of the stems before placing in clean water, cut a further incision lengthways up the stem, creating a 'V' shape, so that the lilacs can drink up more water. When choosing which stems either to buy or to pick, choose ones where the flowers have already opened as they will last the longest. Those that are in bud when cut do not, surprisingly, last as long.

◯ **PRESENTATION** Ideally presented as a large bunch to sit in a vase or jug of water, lilacs also look good in a bouquet or arrangement. These flowers should not be kept out of water for long as they will fade quickly. Lilacs look prettiest when the green leaves have been stripped away, leaving just the wonderful blossom on display.

As with so many flowers, lilacs have a deep-rooted history that originates in ancient mythology. Lilac's name is said to come from a Greek myth involving the god of forests, groves and fields, Pan, who was in love with a nymph named Syringa (the Latin name for lilac). When he was chasing her through the forest, she turned herself into a lilac shrub to disguise herself. The lilac has continued to be associated with love and romance throughout history, particularly first love. With the early bloom of lilac, and the fact that the god Pan was a deity of both spring and fertility, it often represents first love, early beginnings and renewal.

Lilac flowers range in colour from white, symbolising purity and innocence (and therefore young love), blue, which suggests tranquillity, violet, meaning spirituality and magenta, representing love and passion.

With their short season of just three weeks, lilacs are often associated with Easter. As their scent is used for its soothing, relaxing and uplifting effects, these flowers are perfect for anyone in need of a pick-me-up.

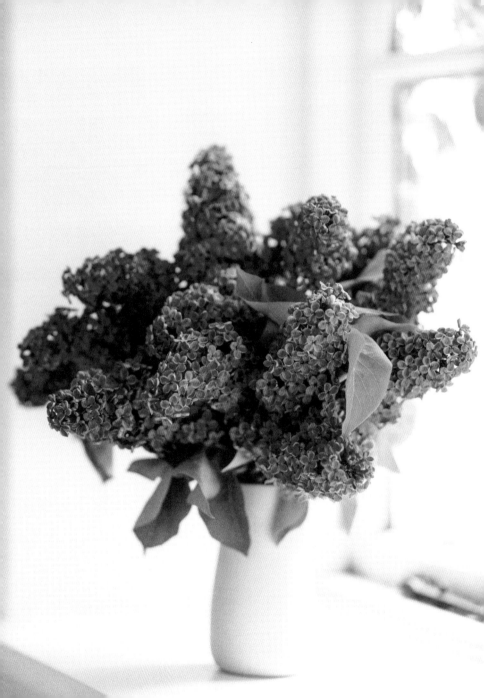

Hellebores

FLOWERING PERIOD
November to April

CARE Trim regularly and refresh water daily. If the flowers wilt, trim the ends again and submerge the whole flower – stalk, sepals and all – in a sink or bucket of very cold water until it comes back to life.

Most importantly, hellebores are winter flowers and like the cold, so won't do well in an overheated room.

PRESENTATION A small hellebore in a terracotta pot makes a wonderful gesture, as does a few lined up in a row. Otherwise, these are welcome additions to an arrangement or bouquet.

TOXIC

The hellebore is also known as the Lentern rose, the Christmas rose, or the snow rose. The Latin genus name *helleborus* comes from a combination of the Greek *helein*, 'to kill', and *bora*, meaning 'food', translating as 'food that kills'. Hellebores contain alkaloids and other chemicals that can lead to poisoning, so don't eat them, no matter how delicious they look!

Hellebores are prized by florists for their elegant, long-lasting winter blooms. Unlike other flowers, their petals are actually sepals, which, unlike petals, stay attached to the plant for a long time and rarely fall off. For this reason, they represent longevity, constancy and strength. As with many things, the durability of this flower depends on how you care for it. Remember that even the most wonderful of friendships and relationships need a lot of care and attention, too.

Hellebores are an ideal token of long-lasting friendship and love. The fact that they flower in winter, a season when moods can be low and we're often in need of cheering up, makes them an even more timely gift.

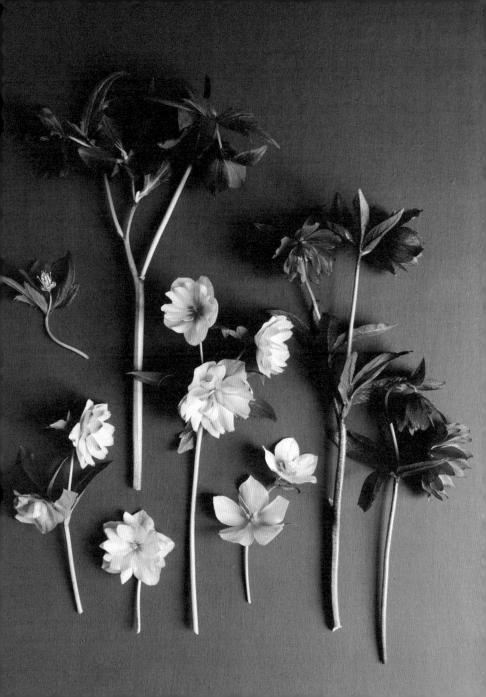

Wallflowers

FLOWERING PERIOD
March to April

CARE These flowers wilt quickly if left out of water for any length of time. As there may be many little branches of flowers opening at different times, cut these off into smaller stems. Trim stems and replace water daily.

PRESENTATION A small posy of wallflowers presented in a jar or small vase makes a simple, pretty gift. Otherwise, these also do well as filler flowers in both arrangements and bouquets.

This plant, originally from Southern Europe, blooms in early spring and has a delightful, sweet scent. Its English name refers to the fact that in the wild it grows in walls and rocks, though it is successfully planted in flower beds by many gardeners. Its formal name, *Cheiranthus*, is made up of the Greek words *cheir*, meaning 'hand', and *anthos*, meaning 'flower', referring to the custom in which flowers are carried to festivals and celebrations, much as they are today at weddings.

Often long and leggy when growing as a plant, the flowers that are nearest the base of the stem open first – you will often find eight or ten separate flowers blooming at the same time.

Although we now think of wallflower as a description for someone who is shy, in floriographical terms, it represents fidelity, faithfulness and lasting beauty – perfect attributes for a symbol of enduring friendship. The simple nature of both the flower and its meaning make it an ideal gesture of companionship.

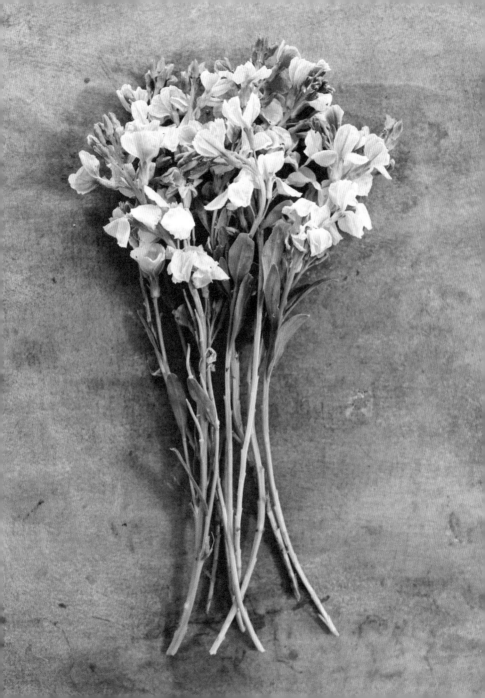

Hydrangeas

FLOWERING PERIOD
June to September

CARE Crush, cut or break woody branches in an upwards motion, leaving a longer cut surface area so that more water can be taken in. While many hydrangeas hold their shape well, particularly when dried, some can wilt quite easily. Unusually, hydrangeas drink from their heads as well as their stems, so it is a good idea to spray them with water to perk them up from time to time. Trim ends regularly and refresh water daily.

PRESENTATION
Hydrangeas look wonderful grouped together or in several bunches. They can also be used at the base of arrangements or bouquets (they are good at holding together a floral structure) and dry very well, too.

The flowers pictured here have been dried.

These large statement flowers are made up of round bundles of tiny flowers all bunched together on one large head. Available to buy in pinks, blues, creams and lilacs during the summer, as autumn approaches, their shades deepen to greens, reds and eventually browns. The different colours traditionally signify different meanings: pink represents heartfelt emotion, blue is for an apology and purple is said to represent the desire to understand someone. They make wonderful dried flowers, as seen here, and are often seen hanging upside down on flower stalls towards the end of autumn.

Hydrangeas are traditionally an emblem of devotion and appreciation. They are particularly significant in Japan. According to legend, the plant came to signify feelings of gratitude and understanding after a Japanese emperor gave them to the family of a girl that he loved but had neglected. He hoped the flowers would atone for his behaviour. Even the appearance of the plant is one that brings to mind the importance of working together. When you look at all the tiny flowers that make one compact form, they resemble individuals that have formed a community to enable them to make a big impact. This show of unity makes them the perfect token to give to someone you value and want to have on your team.

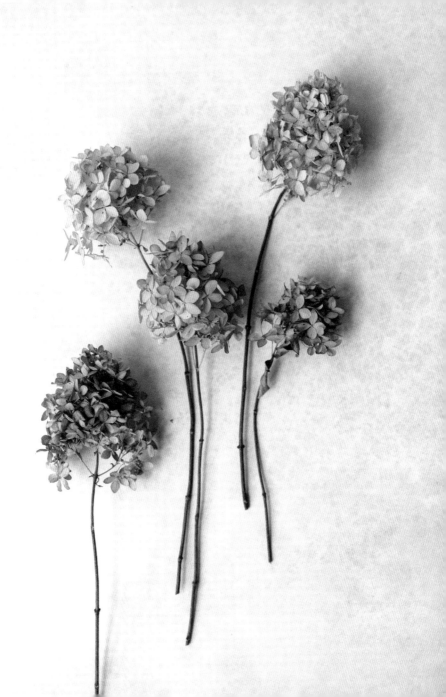

Pansies

⊕ **FLOWERING PERIOD**
May to October

⊕ **CARE** Trim ends regularly
and refresh water daily.

⊗ **PRESENTATION** As
pansies are smaller flowers
with shorter stems, they
tend to look best either in a
small glass jar or at the very
bottom of arrangements.
They also make wonderful
pressed flowers.

With flat, open faces turned gently upwards,
and soft, velvety petals, pansies mean 'keep me
in your thoughts'. The French word for this flower,
pensée, translates as 'thought', which further
reinforces this flower's request to be kept in the
beholder's mind.

Pansies come in many colours, and some
of these have specific meanings: in particular
yellow is associated with happiness and blue
with trustworthiness. The pansy was very
popular with the Victorians, who believed it
embodied virtues such as concern, friendship
and compassion. A token for a friend would
often include pansies and today it still makes
a similar gesture. It is the perfect flower to give
to a dear friend if you would like them to hold
you in their thoughts, or to let them know
that you are thinking of them.

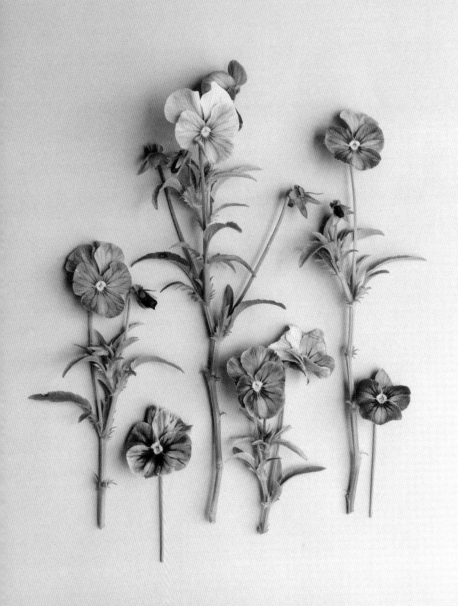

Geraniums

🏵 **FLOWERING PERIOD**
June to November

⊕ **CARE** Trim ends regularly
and refresh water daily
if using as a cut flower.
If in pots, make sure the
soil is kept moist, but not
overwatered.

💍 **PRESENTATION**
Geraniums are most
often presented planted in
terracotta pots (or similar)
but they can also make good
cut flowers to work into an
arrangement.

The geranium, with its brightly coloured flowers and cheerful nature, is a common sight in window boxes and on kitchen windowsills. The oak-leaved geranium that's also known as a *perlagonium*, which we are concerned with here, was designated as the emblem of true friendship in reference to the strength and duration of the oak tree.

The geranium is widely used in aromatherapy to help relieve symptoms such as depression, anxiety, discontent and stress. It is also used to heal poor relationships, which is all the more appropriate when one considers its symbolic meaning of friendship.

Geraniums are the perfect token to give to a dear friend who you will always be there for, or to someone who has been there for you.

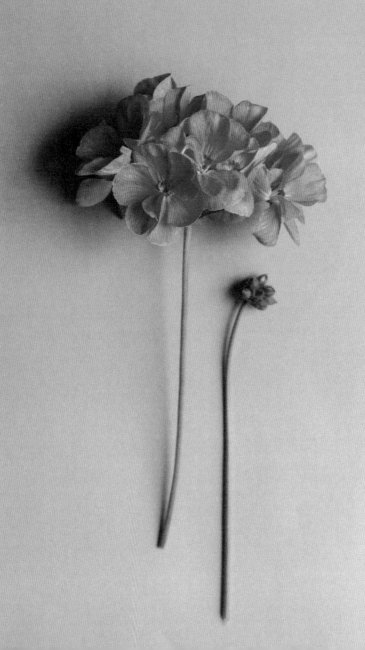

Alstroemerias

FLOWERING PERIOD
May to September

CARE Trim ends regularly
and refresh water daily.
Lasts particularly well as
a cut flower.

PRESENTATION
Alstroemerias look
good in both bouquets
and arrangements.

TOXIC

The alstroemeria looks rather like a miniature lily and comes in a variety of different colours including white, yellow, pink, orange and dark purple. A very long-lasting flower, alstroemeria symbolises fortune, prosperity, longevity and a powerful bond with another person. It is indicative of devotion, friendship and mutual support. Even its leaves grow upside down, twisting out from the stem rather like the twists and turns one might find in a friendship or on the road to success.

Within the range of colours available, white flowers are symbolic of strength, support and love, pink represents playfulness and love and yellow is vibrant and fun – all desirable traits in a friendship or relationship.

Alstroemerias are the perfect flower to give to someone to let them know you've got their back, or to thank them for being your rock. They could also be given to a friend or partner with whom you have enjoyed some luck or success.

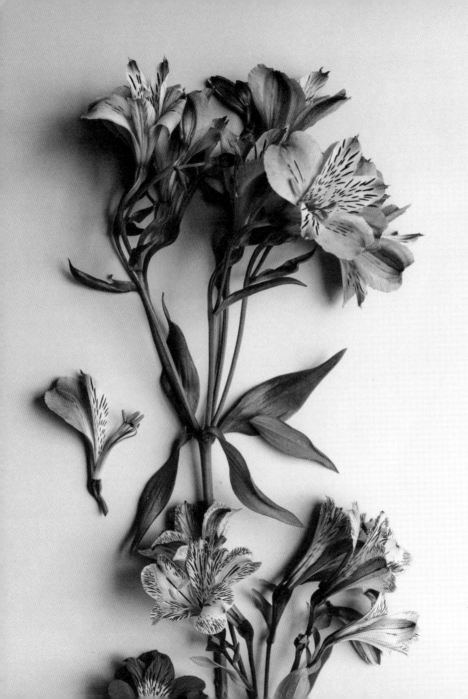

Strawflowers

✿ FLOWERING PERIOD
June to October

⊕ CARE If keeping in a vase,
trim ends regularly and
refresh water daily, being
careful that the stems do
not get mouldy. If drying,
hang upside down in a dark,
dry place.

⚇ PRESENTATION
Strawflowers look great
by themselves in a bunch
or can be worked into
fresh flower arrangements
and bouquets. They are
wonderful dried and make
unusual and pretty additions
to seasonal wreaths.

⚠ TOXIC

These delightful and cheery paper flowers come
in a mix of colours including deep reds, bright
pinks, pale pastel yellows and oranges as well as
creams and silvery whites. Sometimes referred to
as paper daisies, these flowers are often associated
with childhood and simple things on account
of their lack of pretension, and it might be for
this reason that they have been overlooked in the
past, though they are now enjoying a revival due
to the popularity of dried flowers.

Traditionally strawflowers are seen as symbols
of agreement, constancy, continual happiness,
health and longevity, which ties in with their
everlasting nature, as they are often used in
dried flower arrangements.

Strawflowers make a wonderful token to give
to someone with whom you have either spent
a lot of happy times or would like to.

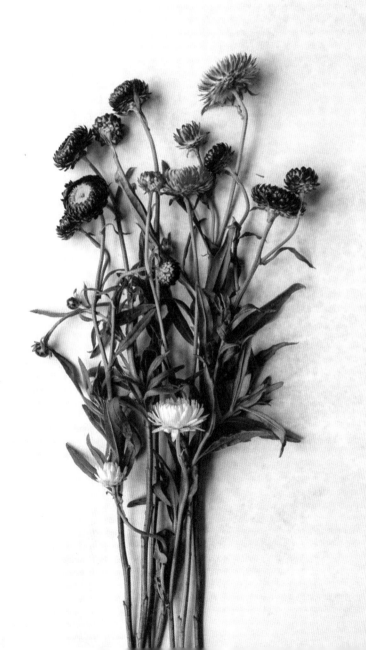

Mistletoe

FLOWERING PERIOD
October to May

CARE Once mistletoe
has been cut it is hard to
preserve, but keep it cool
(or no more than average
room temperature) and it
should last around seven
to ten days. If it looks a
bit dry, try spritzing it with
cold water.

PRESENTATION
Most commonly seen sold
in bunches and hung indoors
in places under which people
can kiss.

TOXIC

Mistletoe, which grows high in leafless trees, appears to have no roots or obvious means by which it can sustain itself with water and nutrients, yet it remains green and produces opaque white berries. Surprisingly able to thrive in these conditions, mistletoe was seen to mean 'I surmount difficulties'.

The practice of kissing under the mistletoe may have begun at the Greeks' Kronia festival, which was held to mark the harvest. The Romans, who celebrated the Saturnalia at around the same time as we now celebrate Christmas, combined disorderly behaviour with mistletoe. And Pliny the Elder noted that the Druids of Gaul also considered mistletoe to be sacred. They believed it helped to cure diseases, protect against evil forces and bring good luck to those who kept it on their person. The Ancient Celts hung mistletoe to ward off bad spirits and to welcome in the New Year.

The Victorians loved to have mistletoe in their homes at Christmas. They decorated their hallways and doorframes with sprigs and introduced the well-known custom of hanging a bunch up high for two people to kiss underneath it. In France it is more customary to do this at

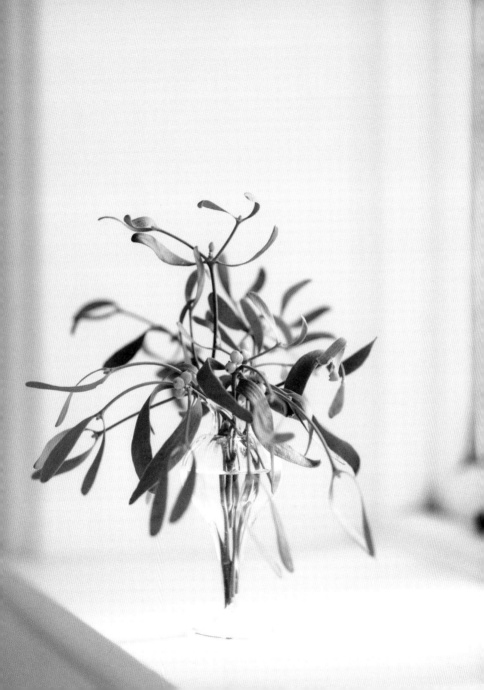

New Year and the French often gift mistletoe to friends to wish them luck in the year ahead.

Give mistletoe to your loved one or carry a bunch to surprise them with, as you steal a kiss from them beneath it. Whatever the celebration, it's the ideal way to wish someone love and good luck in the coming year.

Stocks

April to October

⊕ CARE Trim stems regularly
and refresh water daily,
especially as stocks can
smell a little like cabbages
if their water is not changed
often enough. Sometimes
the tops of these flowers can
seem a little ragged. If they
appear to be thinner at the
end, chop the top section of
the bloom down to the part
where the flowers are
thicker and denser.

⚲ PRESENTATION Stocks
mix well with most other
flowers, and their sturdy
stems lend themselves to
padding out both bouquets
and arrangements. A vase of
mixed stocks also looks
very pretty.

The stock, with its delicious, clove-like scent,
is the emblem of lasting beauty, contentment
and happiness. It is available in a great variety
of colours, ranging from creamy white and pale
pinks through to deep burgundy shades.

The sturdy stems and long-lasting blooms
make stocks wonderful on their own, but they
are also a happy friend to many other flowers.
It's a little bit like the person you want to have
at your party because you know they will give
off cheerful vibes, look good and get on with
everyone else too. For this reason, stocks are
a lovely gesture to a good friend, as a thank you
or just to let them know you appreciate them.

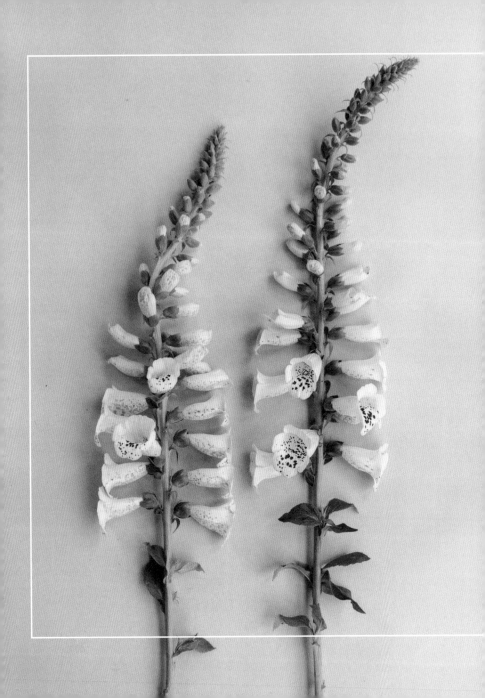

Flowers
for
<u>Success</u>

Lily of the valley

FLOWERING PERIOD
April to May

CARE These very small flowers do not last long out of water, so add them to arrangements and bouquets at the last possible moment. Keep stems trimmed and change water daily if they are in a vase.

PRESENTATION Lily of the valley is so pretty and fragrant that it makes a joyful bunch of flowers in its own right. Presented as cut flowers in a vase or potted up in terracotta vessels (or similar) are both beautiful ways to bring the scent indoors. It is also lovely in bridal or bridesmaid bouquets; Grace Kelly carried a simple bouquet of lily of the valley on her wedding day.

TOXIC

This tiniest and most delicate of plants has a powerful meaning that belies its size.

If you search for the symbolism of lily of the valley, you are repeatedly brought back to the meaning 'a return to happiness', which makes it the perfect flower to give in troubled times as a symbol of hope and the promise of the future to come.

Lily of the valley typically flowers when hard frosts and freezing weather are behind us, heralding the arrival of warmer and happier times. In pagan belief, they were the special flower of Ostara, the Norse goddess of dawn.

The French name for lily of the valley is *muguet* and in France they are a symbol for May Day, when lovers present each other with sprigs of the flower. The tradition is believed to have begun with Charles IX, who was given lily of the valley as a token of luck and prosperity for the coming year. He gave the same floral offering to ladies of his court every year. At the beginning of the twentieth century, lilies were sold on May Day as a symbol of spring, hard work and good harvests.

Lily of the valley is the perfect present to wish someone good luck and success.

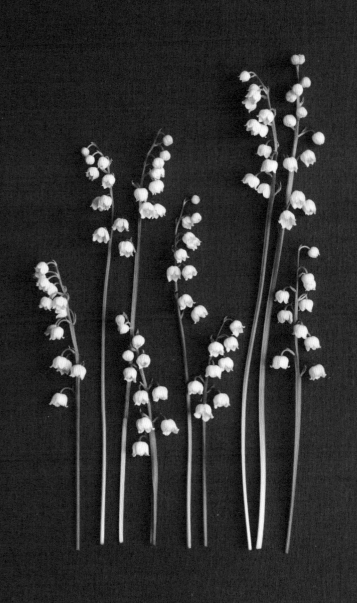

Honesty

✿ FLOWERING PERIOD
Everlasting

⊕ CARE Keep the dried
pods away from damp
and any possible mould
during the winter months
and they should last for
more than a year.

⚬ PRESENTATION These
pods look good grouped
together; they are also
particularly effective in
dried wreaths.

*The plant pictured here
is dried.*

The honesty plant goes through several
different stages during the course of a year. In
spring it produces small flowers on long stems
and in summer it transforms into a deep-green
seed pod. It is most prized among florists in its
final state in autumn, when the pod has dried
out and it takes on a translucent, silvery hue
with a texture a little like crepe paper. For this
reason, honesty is sometimes known as lunaria,
since its colour is similar to the moon. It is also
known as the satin flower, the silver dollar plant
and the money plant.

While honesty is associated with the very
meaning its name represents – honesty – as
well as sincerity, it also has strong associations
with money and luck, hence its other names.
It was believed that the way to encourage
money into one's life was to place a seed from
the honesty plant in the bottom of a candlestick,
put a green candle on top of it and then burn the
candle right down to the end. Another, simpler,
way was to carry a seed of the plant in your
purse or pocket.

Given honesty's strong association with money,
it's an ideal gift for someone starting a new business
venture or hoping to bring some financial
success into their life.

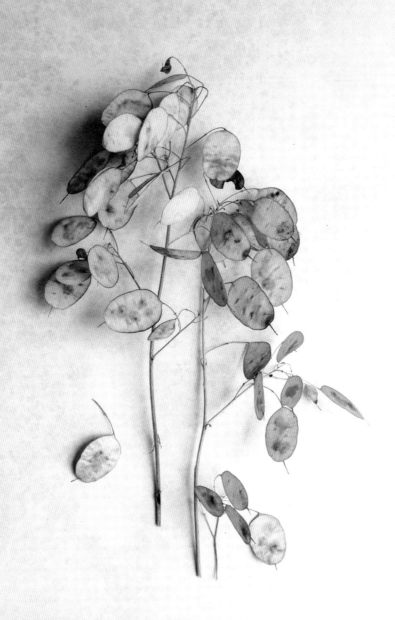

Nicotiana

FLOWERING PERIOD
June to September

CARE Trim ends regularly
and refresh water daily.

PRESENTATION
Nicotiana adds an
ideal floaty element to
both arrangements and
bouquets, but it is fragile,
so be careful when
handling the stems
and heads.

TOXIC

This pretty and delicate flower is a relative of the tobacco plant. Easy to admire for its star-shaped, tubular flowers alone, it was held sacred by some Native American tribes. They believed that smoking the nicotiana plant allowed them to communicate effectively with spirits, while others thought that throwing nicotiana into the water at the beginning of a water journey would appease the water spirit and ensure safe travels.

So, nicotiana is an appropriate flower to give to someone embarking on a new journey or project to wish them luck for a successful venture.

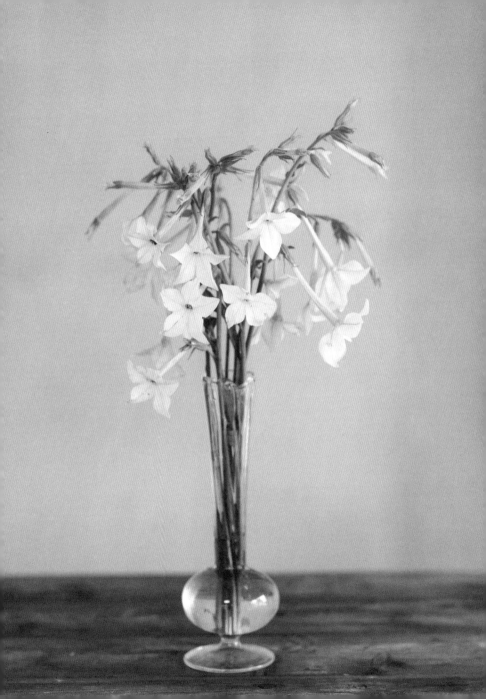

Foxgloves

FLOWERING PERIOD
June to September

CARE Trim the ends
regularly and refresh
water daily.

PRESENTATION
Ideally presented as a large
bouquet to sit in a big jug
of water, foxgloves look
good in both bouquets
and arrangements. Two
colours together can look
particularly pretty.

TOXIC

There are few sights more spellbinding than a field or glen full of foxgloves on a balmy summer's evening. This enchanting flower's name has its origins in early English. An Anglo-Saxon legend tells how sympathetic fairies gave Reynard (the fox) foxglove blossoms to wear on his toes to muffle his approach to his prey.

Foxgloves attract lots of energy in nature – as well as being a food source for moths and butterflies, foxgloves are intoxicating for bees. If we see flower meanings as being not just about the flower itself, but about the energy that they encourage, then the foxglove represents so much more than just its beauty and mythical appeal to fairies. It can be seen as a symbol of productivity and successful teamwork, so makes the perfect present for anyone starting a new job or project. Because of its charm, the foxglove lures in insects, hummingbirds, and good energy. By bringing that energy into the home, they can encourage a desire to give, connect and be engaged.

Foxgloves are perfect to mark the beginning of a new project or job, celebrate a new home, or inspire energy and productivity.

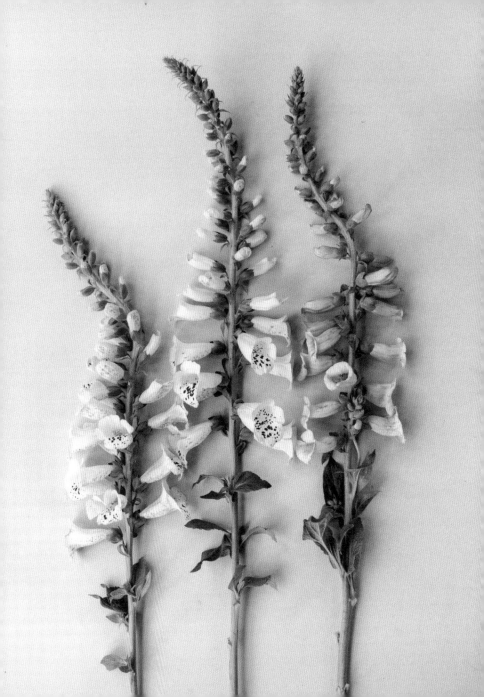

Dogwood

FLOWERING PERIOD
May

CARE Trim ends regularly
and refresh water daily.

PRESENTATION
Dogwood flowers sit on
delicate, curving branches
that make them very useful
for both bouquets and
arrangements. They also
look wonderful when scooped
up and placed on their own
in a large vase or jug.

TOXIC

There are few trees prettier than a dogwood
in full bloom. Its flowering period is short lived,
but the tiny flowers that it produces are so beautiful
that it is worth seeking out. In order to reveal
the flowers, some florists pinch off some of the
leaves surrounding them to help focus the eye
on the blooms themselves, while others prefer
to keep the branches intact. Either way, it is
a beautiful flower to give.

It is said that if you put some sap from the dogwood
tree on a handkerchief on Midsummer's Eve and
carry it with you everywhere, then you will be
granted any wish. Others believe that carrying
a piece of the wood or leaves of a dogwood will
offer the person carrying it protection. Both
these folklores suggest that dogwood is a lucky
flower that will bring success to the recipient.

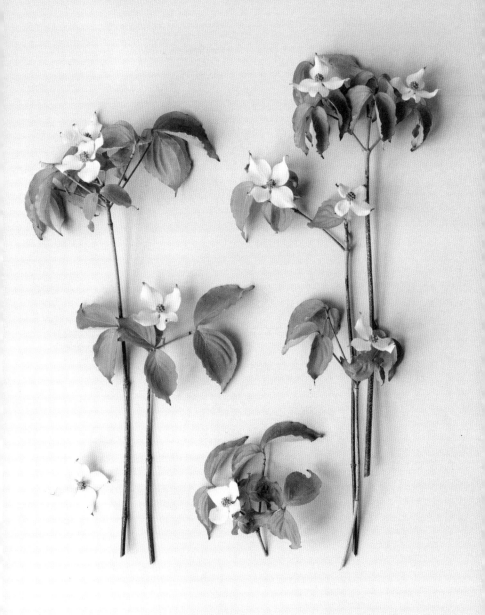

Chrysanthemums

FLOWERING PERIOD
October to December

CARE Chrysanthemums do not particularly like being cut with metal tools. Break flowers to their desired length by hand. Trim stems regularly and change water daily.

PRESENTATION Ideally presented as a bunch to fill a ceramic vase or jug of water, or as a bouquet tied with a naturally dyed silk ribbon. Chrysanthemums are long, leggy plants, but sit best and last longest when cut relatively short.

Chrysanthemums, with their perfectly formed pom-pom flower heads, come into their own in late autumn. Their meanings are rooted in Japanese and Chinese history – the Japanese considered the orderly unfolding of the chrysanthemum's petals to be a symbol of its perfection and a source of its calming energy. They were also the symbol of the Chinese Emperor, and golden flowers in particular are still seen as lucky.

Chrysanthemums are also known to have significant healing properties. They are said to reduce inflammation and nerves, and the drinking of chrysanthemum tea has become increasingly popular.

Common attributes ascribed to them include friendship, longevity, joy, optimism, rest, power and protection, making them versatile gifts. Buddhists use chrysanthemums in offerings due to their powerful yang energy and believe the flower brings luck into the home. Yang energy is bright and positive energy in feng shui and is signalled in bright sounds, bold colours, lights and, as in this case, an upward-moving energy.

Given their varied meanings, chrysanthemums are tokens of good luck and have all the positive attributes of power, wealth and protection.

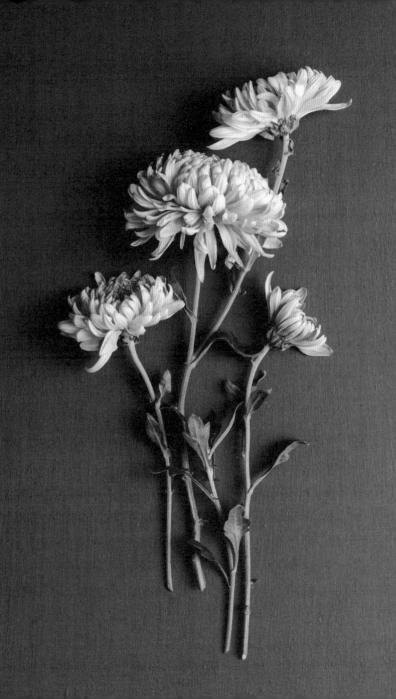

Hollyhocks

⊕ **FLOWERING PERIOD**
June to August

⊕ **CARE** Trim ends regularly
and refresh water daily.

PRESENTATION
Given their height,
hollyhocks sit well at the
back of arrangements,
though you will probably
have to cut them a little
shorter before using
them, depending on the
size of the arrangement.

These tall, thin, beautiful plants are most often
seen alongside country paths and in traditional
cottage gardens, but they also make good cut
flowers. When situated in gardens, hollyhocks
stand proud, towering high and reaching for the
skies. Given the energy that they exude, it is no
surprise that they are an emblem of ambition
and striving, but also of fruitfulness (perhaps
on account of all those endeavours they have
been making to reach upwards).

Hollyhocks make a good present for someone
about to start a new venture, to encourage hard
work, success and maybe even a little bit of
good luck, too.

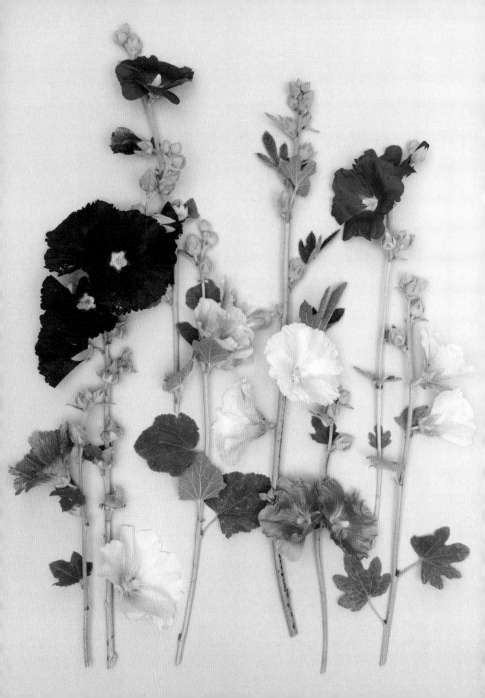

Fritillary

FLOWERING PERIOD
March to April

CARE Trim ends regularly
and refresh water daily to
keep these delicate blooms
going for as long as possible.

PRESENTATION A small
bunch of *fritillaria* in a simple
vase looks pretty, and they
add a perfect wispy element
to arrangements and
bouquets alike.

There are many types of fritillary, but it is the delicate *Fritillaria meleagris*, more commonly known as snake's head fritillary, which we are concerned with here. Even this one variety has a number of names, including chess flower, chequered lily and snake's head lily, while *fritillaria* itself comes from the Latin *frittilus*, meaning 'dice box'. A lot of names for such a relatively small flower. The pattern of the snake's head fritillary doesn't just resemble the chequered pattern of dice, but also chessboards, and so the theme of games, all of which involve an element of luck and desire for success, springs to mind when looking at this tiny flower.

Their connotations as a flower for success are all the more appropriate when you consider the symbolism surrounding the snake, which they so closely resemble. The snake shedding its skin represents transformation, healing and renewal, and a bunch of these flowers would be an appropriate gesture for someone recovering from a period of ill health, restarting a business or switching career.

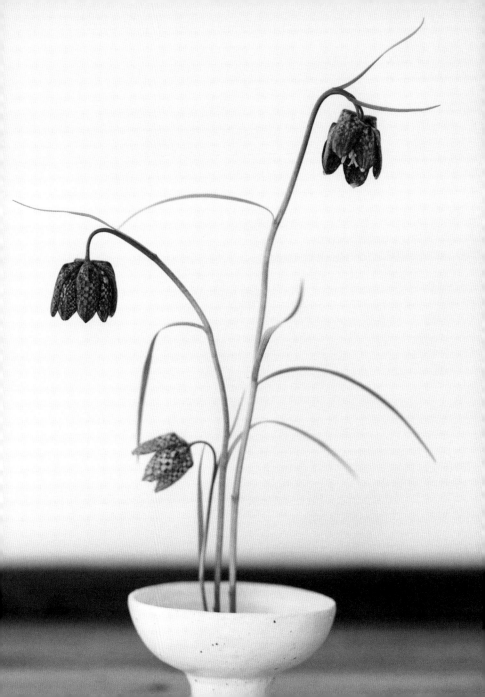

Amaryllises

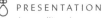

FLOWERING PERIOD
November to March

CARE Amaryllises are sometimes sold with the buds still closed and these will open up over a period of several days. If you are in a hurry for them to open, try cutting the stems a little shorter and putting them in slightly warm water, possibly near a source of heat like a radiator. Amaryllises last longer than many flowers and if properly cared for, with ends trimmed regularly and water changed daily, they can last for up to two weeks.

PRESENTATION
Amaryllises have particularly long, thick stems and stand upright on their own with the need for only a little support. They look good paired with seasonal foliage such as pine or berried branches. Amaryllises also look good potted up as bulbs.

TOXIC

Amaryllises are large, striking flowers grown indoors from bulbs and brighten any windowsill or shelf during the dull and dark days of winter. The amaryllis commonly means determination, beauty and love. The Victorians associated it with strength and resolve because of its height and sturdiness.

The name amaryllis originates from the Greek myth of Amaryllis and Alteo. A young maid named Amaryllis fell in love with a shepherd, Alteo. He was strong and attractive and had a deep love of flowers. To learn how to win his affection, Amaryllis visited the Oracle at Delphi for advice. On the Oracle's orders, Amaryllis stood in front of Alteo's house for thirty nights, piercing her heart with a golden arrow. On the thirtieth night, a beautiful flower grew from her blood and Alteo fell in love with her. Amaryllis can also signify success, therefore, and the flowers are good as a gift to celebrate hard-won achievements.

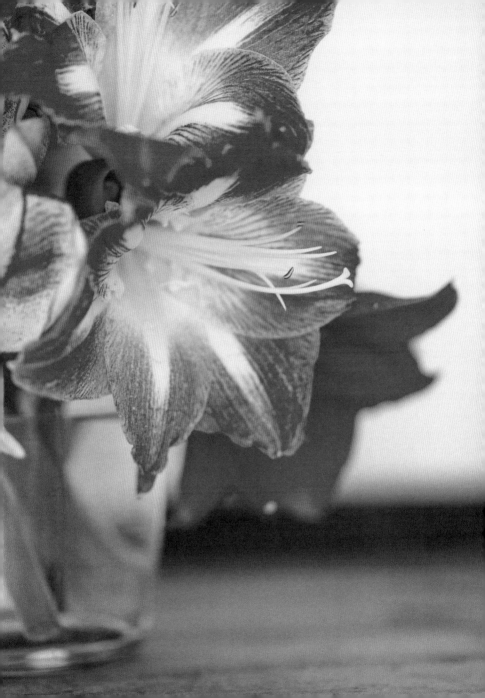

Narcissi

⊕ **FLOWERING PERIOD**
February to April

⊕ **CARE** Trim stems regularly
and change water daily to
ensure a longer lifespan.

⊗ **PRESENTATION** A simple
bunch of narcissi, either of
one type or a variety, makes
a lovely, inexpensive gift.
They can also be added to
bouquets and arrangements.
Narcissi bulbs potted up,
in an old terracotta pot or
stoneware bowl, look lovely
and last up to a week.

There are many types of narcissi showing
off their cheerful yellow blooms in springtime.
Like the daffodil (see page 159), they emerge
in time for Easter celebrations, but they draw
their name and meaning from a story in
Ovid's *Metamorphoses*. The story of Echo
and Narcissus tells of a young nymph called
Echo falling in love with beautiful young man,
Narcissus. He rejects her advances but is punished
by the goddess Nemesis for leading Echo on and
then rejecting her as she causes him to fall in love
with his own reflection. He is so besotted with
this image of himself that he is unable to leave
the pool and eventually dies of starvation.

In spite of the sad ending to this tale, the
narcissus has been taken as a symbol of self-love,
an attribute that has been useful to many who
wish to succeed, giving them the confidence
necessary to achieve success. A bunch of narcissi
makes a wonderful gift for someone taking exams,
setting out on a fresh venture or embarking on
a new beginning.

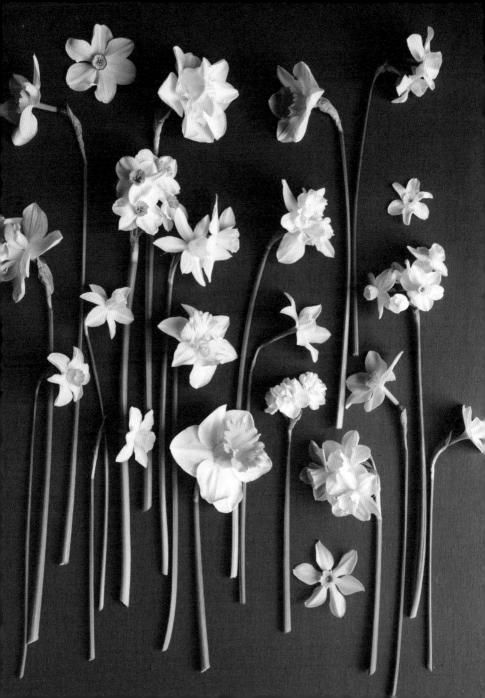

Primroses

FLOWERING PERIOD
February to April

CARE Keep the stems on these little flowers trimmed, but only in very tiny amounts given their small size. Change water daily.

PRESENTATION Not really suitable for inclusion in bouquets or arrangements because of their small size, primroses look best in a small glass or jar as a simple gesture. They also make lovely pressed flowers.

TOXIC

The primrose has many associations and is said to be the flower of youth, birth and sweetness as well as a symbol of safety and protection in Celtic folklore. In ancient times it was placed on the doorstep to encourage fairy folk to bless the house and anyone living in it, and it was also said that if you ate the blooms of the primrose you would see a fairy. It was thought to hold the keys to heaven and so was considered sacred by the ancient Celts.

The primrose was highly prized by the Celtic Druids in particular and its abundance in woods, hedgerows and pastures made it easily collectible. Primroses were often carried by the Druids during certain Celtic rituals as a protection from evil. It was also seen as a flower of love and bringer of good luck and was the symbol of the first day of spring laid across thresholds to celebrate May Day.

A small bunch of primroses makes the perfect good luck gift.

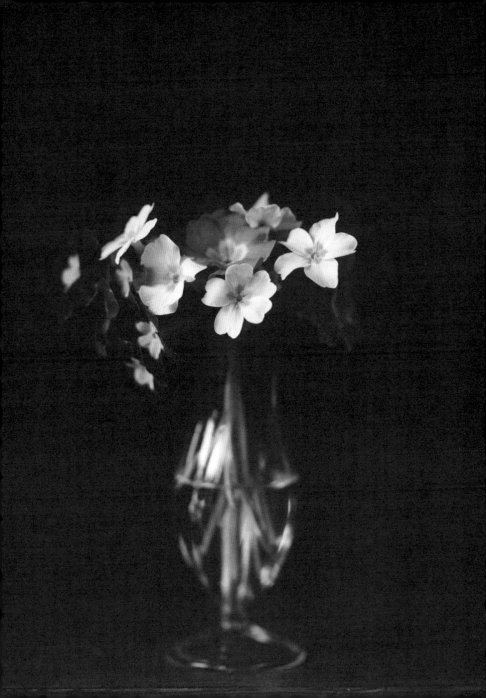

Peonies

FLOWERING PERIOD
May to June

CARE Trims ends regularly and refresh water daily. Peony blossoms open extremely quickly, so choose ones that are still in bud if you want them to last for a long time – if you squeeze the bud it should be soft to the touch like a marshmallow.

PRESENTATION These beautiful flowers work well as a focal bloom in almost every kind of bouquet or arrangement. They are also lovely as abig bunch in a vase, or even as a single stem in a bottle.

Almost everyone loves these plump, fluffy balls of petals, sometimes referred to as the 'rose without thorns', and they are possibly the most requested flower by brides due to their prettiness.

The peony is often associated with devotion, but it has been a favourite in China for many centuries, where it is seen as a symbol of luck, happiness, fortune and wealth. It is often seen on both Chinese porcelain and screen paintings, and its name *Sho Yu* means 'most beautiful'.

If you combine the unrivalled beauty of this flower with its associations (both its traditional meaning of devotion and the Eastern interpretation of luck, success and happiness), then there is hardly a more appropriate flower for a wedding bouquet. Giving peonies as a present is the perfect way to wish someone good fortune, joy and prosperity.

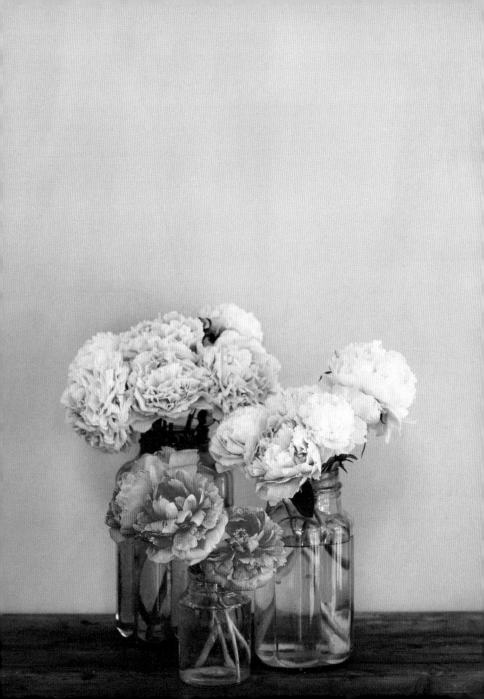

Sunflowers

FLOWERING PERIOD
July to September

CARE Sunflowers last particularly well, providing you trim the ends regularly and refresh water daily.

PRESENTATION It depends on which size and variety you use, but generally larger sunflowers look best bunched together in a large glass vase or similar.

The sunflower is perhaps the boldest and cheeriest of all the flowers with its big, open face and petals standing proud on a tall, thick stem. Traditionally yellow in colour, more recent varieties have included subtle brown colours and even shades of red.

According to Ancient Greek legend, a nymph named Clytie fell in love with the sun god Apollo. Although Clytie was beautiful, Apollo did not love or acknowledge her. After nine days of hopeless devotion, the nymph transformed herself into a sunflower and constantly turned towards the sun so she could see her beloved Apollo in his bright and beautiful chariot.

When planted in the ground, and absorbing as much sun as possible, the sunflower rises high above all other flowers, showing its lofty ambitions and desire to succeed. Some can grow as high as three metres tall, so it is no surprise that this flower is associated with ambition, good luck, lofty thoughts, opportunity, pride, strength and wealth. It is the perfect token to give to someone who is starting out on a new venture or taking exams – someone who likes the bold and beautiful!

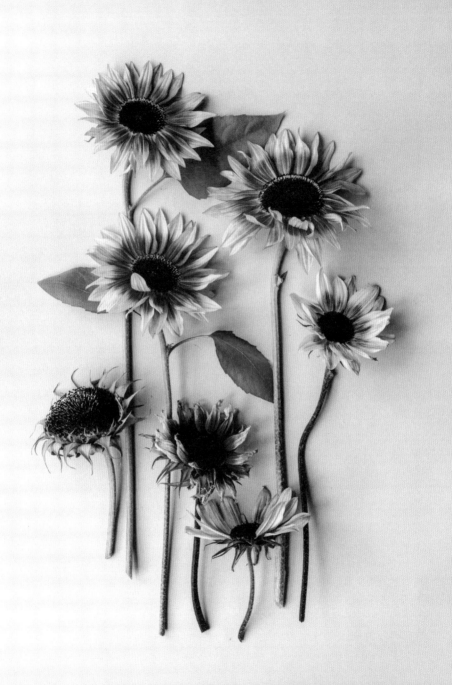

Nasturtiums

✿ FLOWERING PERIOD
July to September

⊕ CARE Trim ends regularly
and refresh water daily.

⚲ PRESENTATION
Nasturtiums look pretty
trailing from a small glass jar
or vase and are also good
flowers for filling gaps in
arrangements.

These small, funnel-shaped flowers grow on delicate vines, yet their nature is anything but dainty. This is a robust flower that will grow anywhere and everywhere.

Their scent is sweet like honey and the spicy leaves add a peppery flavour to salads while the blooms are prized as a cut flower. Available in a range of colours including reds and pinks through to the more traditional oranges and yellows, and even white, they look good weaving through arrangements, adding a lightness of touch to any piece.

The botanist Carl Linnaeus, who gave the nasturtium its scientific name, *Tropaeolum*, thought that the flame-orange flower looked rather like a blood-stained warrior's helmet that had been pierced by a spear. Nasturtiums are known as a symbol of conquest and victory in battle and, with all their positive energy and persistent nature, they make an ideal gift for someone looking for luck and success in any area of life or any venture.

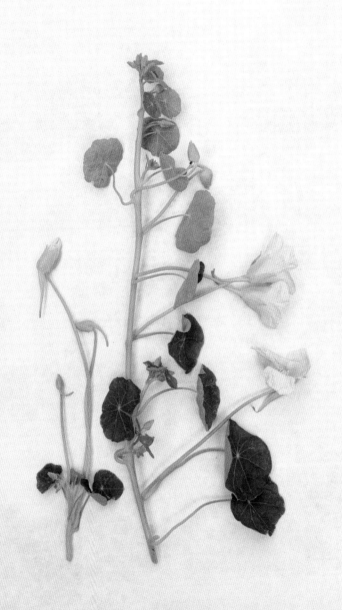

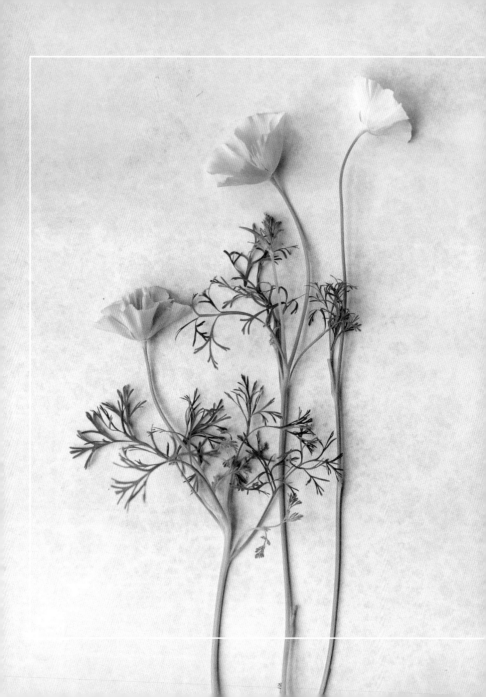

Flowers

to

Console

Anemones

FLOWERING PERIOD
March to May

CARE Their soft stems make them delicate, so handle with care to ensure they do not snap. Trim ends regularly and refresh water daily. Anemones continue to grow in the vase after they have been cut.

PRESENTATION
Lovely grouped together in a vase, as a colourful bunch to brighten up a room, or as part of an arrangement. With their black centres, these flowers also add a hint of sophistication to a piece that might otherwise have a cottagey feel to it and mix well with softer flowers. There are also white anemones with green centres if you are looking for a more delicate overall effect.

TOXIC

These beautiful, delicate flowers were introduced to the rest of the world from Greece in the sixteenth century, and their meaning can be traced back to Greek mythology and a tale recounted in Ovid's *Metamorphoses*. Ovid tells the story of Aphrodite, the Greek goddess of love, who fell for a handsome hunter named Adonis. Their love was short-lived as he was injured by a wild boar and died in Aphrodite's arms. Red anemones were said to have sprung up where droplets of his blood fell. They are said to represent the fleeting nature of love.

The name anemone comes from the Greek word *anemos* meaning 'wind', and their petals appear to dance in the breeze. Their lives are also short and fleeting like a breath of wind.

Anemones make a fitting tribute after the loss of a loved one, or as consolation for something else that was dear but has been lost.

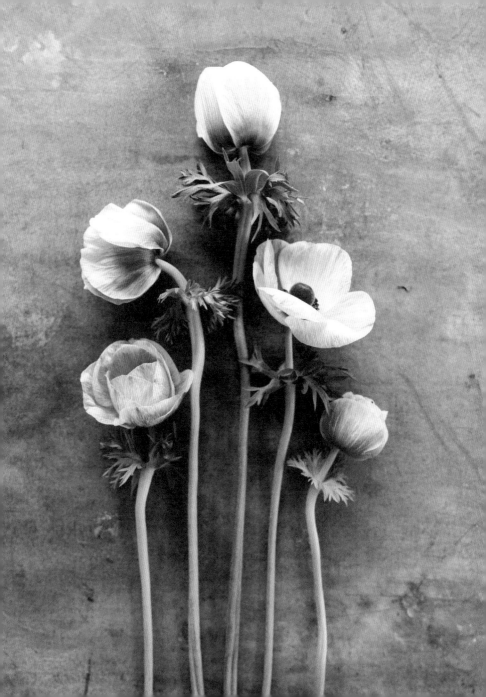

Scabious

FLOWERING PERIOD
June to October

CARE Trim ends regularly
and refresh water daily.

PRESENTATION These
flowers work well in both
big and small arrangements
and bouquets, adding a
floaty touch wherever
they are included.

Scabious is often referred to as the pincushion flower, as its centre looks rather like a good place to keep your pins and needles. Traditionally, scabious is said to have very sad meanings, such as unfortunate love, 'I have lost all', and is associated with widowhood. For this reason, it is also sometimes known as mournful widow.

This makes scabious a fitting flower to give to someone who is mourning the death of their life partner, and it could even be included in a funeral wreath. While it is hard to imagine such a pretty flower having such a sad meaning, it does allow you to give a beautiful, natural and imaginative choice of flower even at a time of loss.

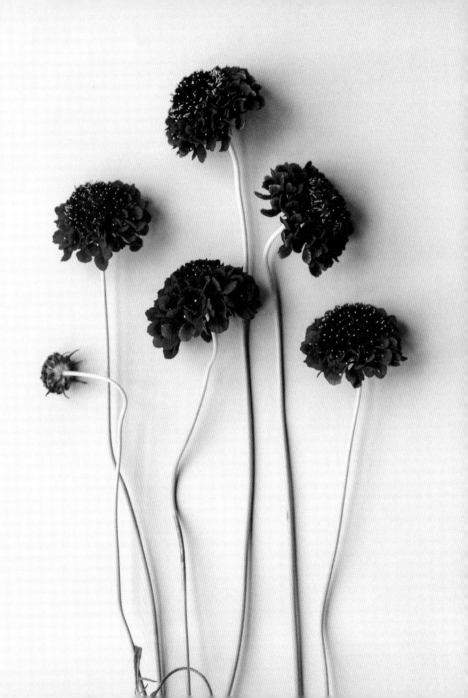

Statice

FLOWERING PERIOD
June to September

CARE If using as a fresh
flower, trim ends regularly
and refresh water daily.

PRESENTATION Statice
looks good in bouquets and
arrangements but it works
particularly well as a dried
flower and adds a wonderful
touch to a wreath.

Statice is also known as sea lavender, on
account of its misty, sea-foam-like appearance.
It is sometimes referred to as limonium, meaning
'meadow', where it is often found growing. The
flowers range from purples and pinks through
to whites, and their frothy appearance adds
a textural element when they are mixed with
other flowers, especially with dried flowers.

Traditionally a symbol of remembrance
and sympathy, statice is a perfect token to give
to someone who has recently suffered a loss.
The fact that this flower dries so well and has
an everlasting quality adds a further layer
of meaning, representing the lasting nature
of our love for those that we have lost.

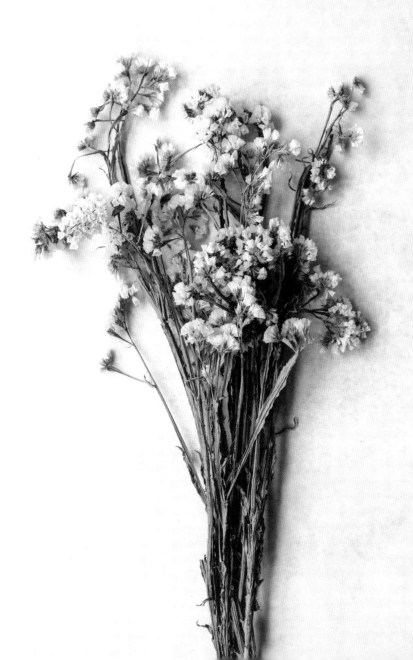

Marigolds

FLOWERING PERIOD
June to October

CARE Trim ends regularly
and refresh water daily.

PRESENTATION
As marigolds are quite
short-stemmed compared
to many other flowers, they
look wonderful presented
in a small glass jar or similar,
but also make good filler
flowers towards the
bottom, or lower, parts
of an arrangement.

Sometimes referred to as 'the herb of the sun', marigolds are cheerful-looking flowers that come in yellows, oranges and even reds, but their vibrancy is at odds with their melancholy meaning. The flower stays open for as long as the sun is shining; at the end of the day it closes tightly shut and its head droops, as if with sadness. The following morning, it is often drenched with dew as it begins to reopen in response to the sunlight. While the marigold symbolises grief and sadness, its reopening in the morning also indicates that happiness will return in time, as sure as the sun will rise.

In Mexico, marigolds play a central part in Día de los Muertos (Day of the Dead) celebrations, where the altar decorations usually include paper marigolds, or freshly cut ones. The celebration honours friends and family that have died, and marigolds are believed to lead the dead souls to the altar.

The sombre meaning of marigolds can be softened by mixing them with other flowers. Pair them with roses to express the bittersweet nature of love or mix with a bloom symbolising friendship, such as geraniums, to tell the recipient that you are thinking of them in their time of distress.

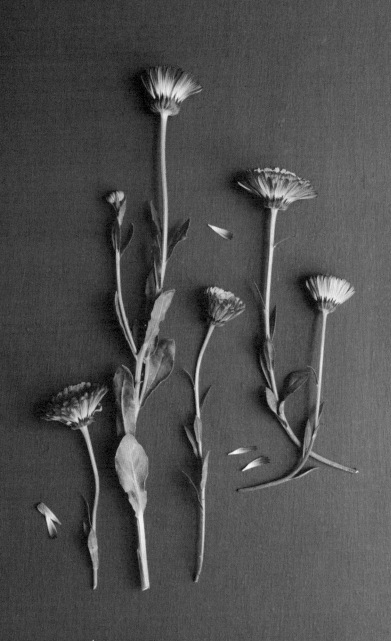

Lupins

CARE Trim ends regularly
and refresh water daily.
These flowers have a short
life span of just a couple
of days.

PRESENTATION A tangle
of multicoloured lupins in
a large vase is a wonderful
sight. Alternatively, they sit
well in arrangements but
die quickly when out of
water and so are not ideal
for hand-held bouquets.

TOXIC

These tall spires of exotic-looking flowers
share their name with the Latin word for wolf,
lupus, in spite of looking more like the plumage
of a bird of paradise. Lupins come in a wide
variety of colours: dark burgundy, deep purple,
white, orange and even pale lemon, but it is pink
lupins that are traditionally most symbolic of
the memories of those who have died.

American First Lady Lady Bird Johnson,
who had a great love of flowers, promoted the
growing of all types of flowers in the central
reservations and by the roadside by order
of the United States Highway Beautification
Act, which is often referred to 'Lady Bird's Bill'.
One result of this is a huge presence of lupins
growing in the wild across Texas.

The lupin stands for imagination, admiration and
happiness. When given as a gift, the lupin, standing
proud and tall, it is said to bring the energy of
inner strength to help the recipient recover from
loss or bereavement. It tells the recipient that
while a loss is terribly sad, in time they will
recover and discover new opportunities.

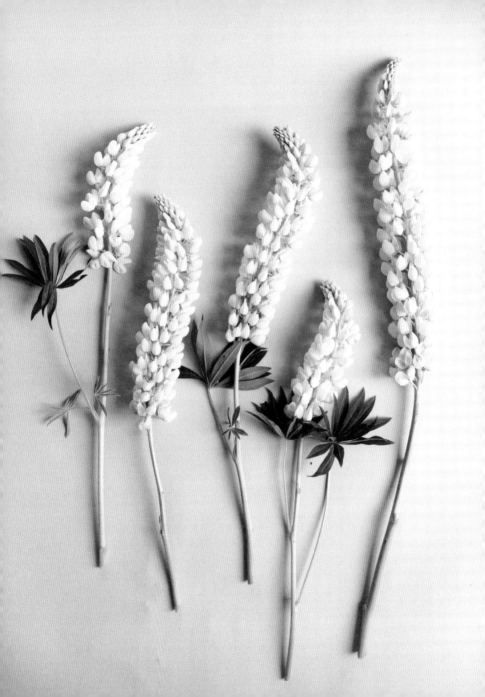

Aquilegia

FLOWERING PERIOD
May to June

CARE Trim stems regularly and refresh water daily to ensure these flowers last well, but take care when handling them as they are very fragile.

PRESENTATION
These delicate flowers sit well in both bouquets and arrangements, their nodding heads giving some movement and a light touch to whatever they are mixed with.

TOXIC

Fully double, nodding flowers sitting on top of stiff stems, aquilegia are sometimes known as Granny's bonnets because of their shape, but in fact they get their name from the Latin *aquila* meaning 'eagle', because the flower is thought to resemble an eagle's foot.

The Greeks and the Persians declared that the eagle was the sun's representative, a symbol of spirit, and associated with the sky god. In early Christianity, the eagle was seen as a sign of hope and strength representing salvation. In the sacred Native American belief of spirit animals, the eagle represents looking at things from a new perspective, being courageous and patient with the present, knowing that the future may hold possibilities not yet seen before the eagle takes flight.

With symbolic meanings for aquilegia including resolution and strength, it was traditionally worn by people for courage. It is a fitting gift for someone who has been grieving or experienced a period of sorrow and is about to spread their wings and begin a new chapter in their lives.

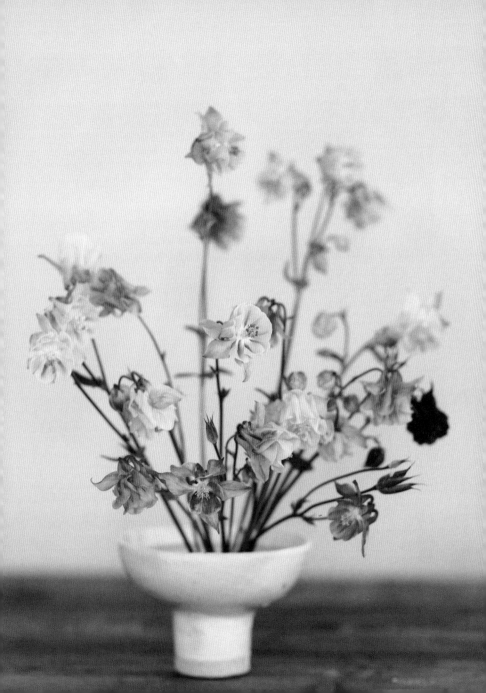

Zinnias

CARE Trim ends regularly and refresh water daily. If well cared for, zinnias have a particularly good vase life of a week or possibly a little longer.

PRESENTATION Zinnias look good on their own in a vase, or in a row of small glass bottles arranged along a windowsill or similar shelf or mantelpiece. They also last well in bouquets and arrangements.

Zinnias were introduced to the West from Mexico more than 200 years ago. In spite of their bright, showy displays, which have a variety of meanings according to their colour, their overall meaning is one of absent friends and remembrance.

Pink zinnias symbolise lasting affection, scarlet ones stand for constancy, white for goodness and yellow for daily remembrance. When the colours are mixed together, they stand for memories of those we have lost. In spite of their sad meaning, a bright bunch of zinnias in mixed colours will hopefully bring consolation to a recipient mourning a loved one.

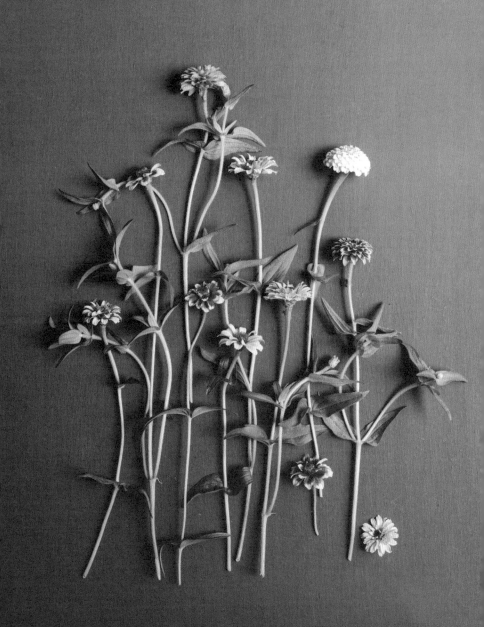

Poppies

CARE If the flowers are
still closed when you receive
them, very gently peel
off the green casing to
reveal the colourful petals.
To extend the life of a poppy,
either scald the end in hot
water or briefly flame its tip
before placing in cold water.
Refresh water daily.

PRESENTATION A mixed
bunch of colourful poppies
in a vase or jar looks very
pretty, but these flowers
also sit well as gestural
blooms in either a bouquet
or an arrangement, though
they may not last as long as
some of the other flowers
they sit alongside.

TOXIC

There are many types of poppy that flower
at different times, from Icelandic poppies in
the early spring to Californian poppies in the
summer. They come in almost every colour
imaginable, from beautiful pastel shades
through to the deep reds we see coveringfields
and recreated so often in art.

John Ruskin wrote that the poppy was the most
delicate of all the blossoms in the field, and like
crumpled pieces of crepe paper on long wavy
stems, they are fragile and fleeting in their beauty.
The Orientalist painters of the nineteenth century
associated them with dreaminess, oblivion and
imagination on account of their opiate qualities,
as can be seen in paintings such as *In the Bey's
Garden* by John Frederick Lewis, *Poppies* by
Eugene Delacroix and *The Oriental Woman*
by Leon Francois Comerre. The red poppies that
filled French fields after the First World War were
said to symbolise the spilled blood of soldiers,
associating them with eternal sleep and the
remembrance of those who have died.

White poppies are a symbol of sympathy,
and so the theme of sleep, death and consolation
continues. These flowers make an ideal token for
someone recently bereaved or suffering a loss.

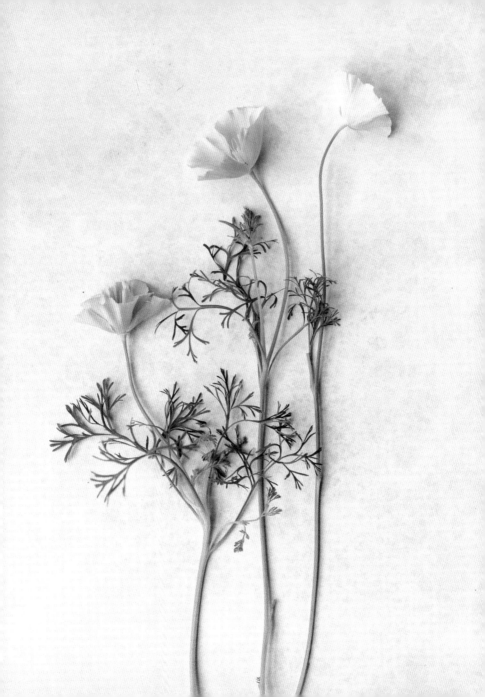

Snowdrops

⊛ FLOWERING PERIOD
January to February

⊕ CARE Keep the stems on
these little flowers trimmed,
but only in very tiny amounts
as they are small. Change
the water they sit in daily.

⚭ PRESENTATION Not
really suitable for bouquets
or arrangements because
they are small, snowdrops
look lovely in a small glass or
jar as a simple gift or token.
Their smell is similar to that
of violets and they bring
a welcome fragrance to a
room. Snowdrops also make
lovely pressed flowers.

*The flowers pictured here
have been pressed.*

The snowdrop is among the very first flowers of the year, blooming in the depths of winter and signalling the hope of more greenery and good things to come in the warmer months ahead. It can also be seen as bringing hope and consolation in darker times, perhaps during a period of unhappiness or after a bereavement.

A small bunch of snowdrops lifts spirits when there are few flowers to be found, signifying that happier times are on their way. Traditionally, a brooch in the shape of a snowdrop was given to someone who had suffered a loss, and snowdrops are often seen on cards for the New Year, sending blessings for the months that lie ahead. They are the perfect symbols of hope and offer consolation in difficult times.

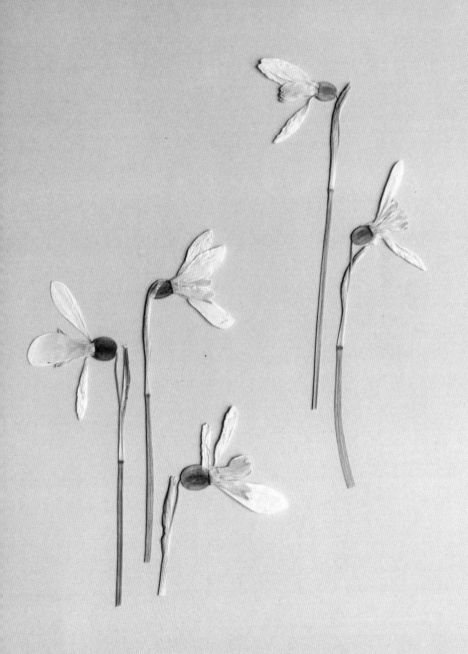

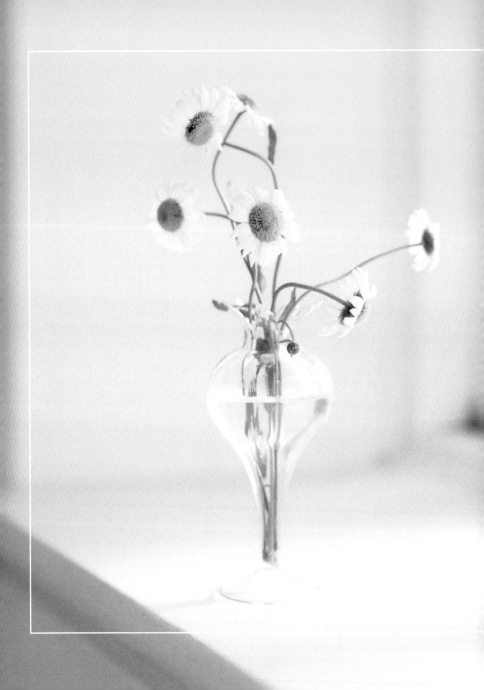

Flowers

to

<u>Celebrate</u>

Iris

FLOWERING PERIOD
May to June

CARE
Trim ends regularly and refresh water daily. When one of the flowers dies, do not discard the whole stem, just remove the dead head as the other flowers will still bloom. This way you get a much longer vase life from your flowers.

PRESENTATION
Irises are such dramatic blooms that just a stem or two in a vase can make a big impact. Alternatively, they sit well in arrangements, either tall towards the back or cut short to sit in the front with other focal flowers.

TOXIC

In Greek mythology, Iris was the messenger of the gods, who used the rainbow as her link between Heaven and Earth. The iris flower comes in a huge array of colours, which is fitting for such a goddess. Its meaning of 'I have a message for you' is equally appropriate.

Within this general theme, many of the colours have more specific meanings – purple flowers bring messages of wisdom and compliments, blue ones symbolise hope and faith, and yellow blooms represent passion.

In classical literature, Iris was often invoked by the gods to deliver all sorts of messages to mortals, as well as other gods, and in medieval iconography the iris was associated with The Annunciation, when the Angel Gabriel informs Mary that she is to bear God's child.

Throughout the ages, the iris has been the symbol of news, so it's an appropriate present to accompany news of some sort, hopefully the kind that involves celebration, such as a new job or a baby on the way.

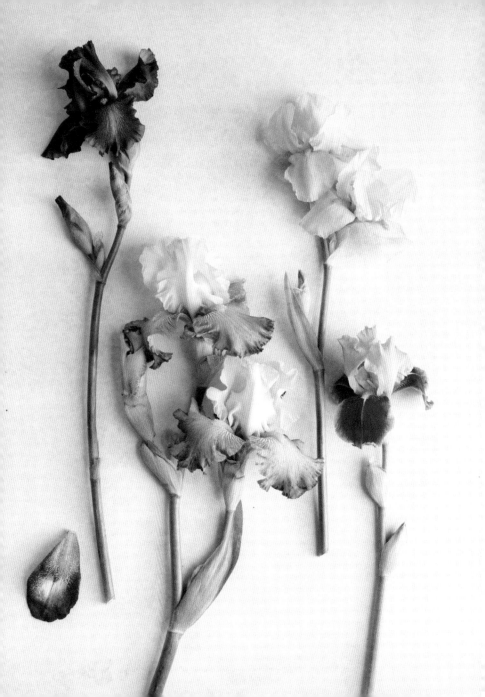

Magnolia

✿ **FLOWERING PERIOD**
March

⊕ **CARE** White magnolia only lasts for up to a day once cut; however, pink lily and saucer-shaped magnolias last well. Keep the woody ends trimmed and refresh the vase water daily.

⚭ **PRESENTATION** Magnolia is so breathtaking that it deserves to be presented on its own, perhaps as a few small branches or one or two big ones – simplicity is key.

Magnolia is one of the most anticipated flowers in the early months of the year, not only due to its stunningly beautiful flowers, but because it signals the drawing to an end of winter. As soon as the magnolia comes out, so do people's cameras, as everyone comes together to celebrate its arrival. It's hard to imagine an Instagram account that doesn't have at least a few images of pretty houses with magnificent magnolia trees outside – it is the ultimate celebration of spring.

Some of the flowers on a magnolia tree look remarkably like candles, perhaps those on a birthday cake, and this only adds to their celebratory nature. A few magnolia branches would make a perfect gift for a celebration, whether a birthday or other joyous occasion, or perhaps even just to mark the end of the long winter months.

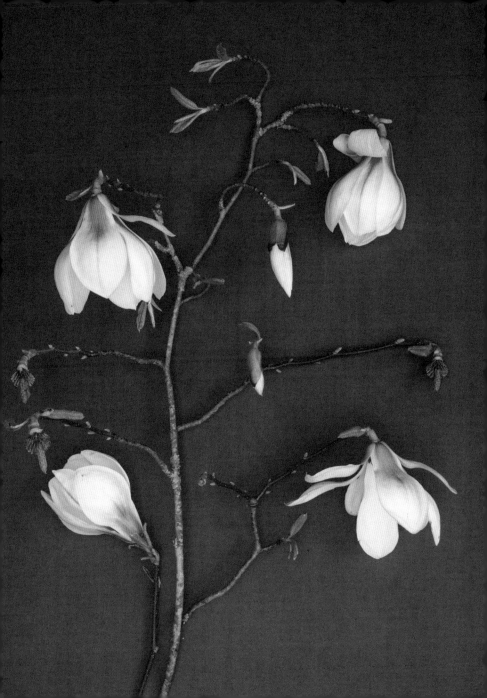

Blossom

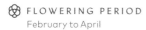

FLOWERING PERIOD
February to April

CARE Trim the woody stems and cut a 'V' shape to ensure water is absorbed. Refresh water daily. Properly cared for, blossoms last well. Once the flowers have finished, don't discard the branches as when left in water they will grow fresh, green shoots.

PRESENTATION
Blossoms can be mixed with almost any flowers. They sit well in an arrangement or a bouquet and also look wonderful bunched together as a single variety in a vase.

The appearance of fluffy blossom in the trees is a welcome sign that spring is on its way.

Such is the popularity and variety of these blooms that many and various meanings and folklores are attached to them. Some say that to find love you should tie a strand of your hair to a cherry blossom tree, others that to guarantee a successful business venture you should climb an almond blossom tree. The ancient Celts, meanwhile, honoured apple blossoms as a symbol of love and used them to decorate their bedchambers.

Blossom is perhaps most famous within the context of Hanami, the Japanese tradition of annual blossom viewings. The Japanese Imperial Court used to celebrate this short-lived but stunning display with annual flower parties and this custom filtered down to all workers and in particular farmers, who would climb mountains to enjoy their lunch under the flowering trees.

Blossom is therefore the perfect celebratory gift to mark a special event or even just the end of winter and the promise of spring to come.

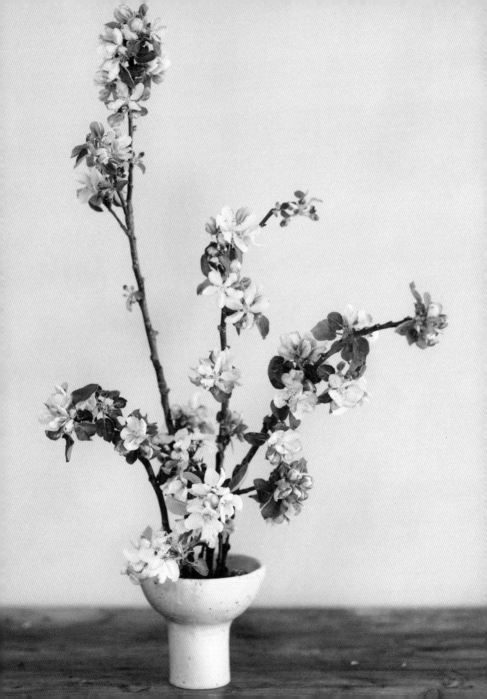

Daisies

FLOWERING PERIOD
June to September

CARE Trim ends regularly
and refresh water daily.

PRESENTATION
If you are using short
daisies picked from outside,
they will have very short
stems and are best either
in a small glass of water,
or as a pressed flower, or
even used to make a daisy
chain. If using longer-
stemmed, cultivated
varieties, they will sit well
in both arrangements and
bouquets or even bunched
together in a vase or jar.

TOXIC

Daisies are among the best known and most-loved flowers, adored by poets and children alike. They are commonly associated with children for a variety of reasons – some believed that a daisy chain wrapped around a child would prevent it from being taken by the fairies. Victorian children would often make a daisy chain for amusement, and a young child might thread daisies into their hair, reflecting a gentle and innocent personality. Other, slightly older, children used a daisy to predict whether or not their beloved returned their affections, picking the petals off one by one and reciting, 'He/She Loves Me, He/She Loves Me Not'.

So strong is the link between daisies and childhood that they make an ideal gift to celebrate the arrival of a new child, invoking all the associations of innocence and joy that they bring.

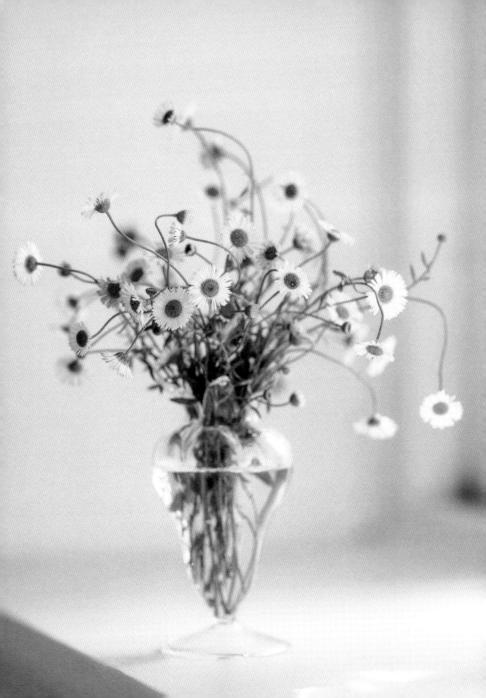

Mimosa

FLOWERING PERIOD
January to April

CARE Trim ends regularly
and refresh water daily.

PRESENTATION Mimosa
adds a cheerful element to
winter bouquets and
arrangements. It also looks
good bunched in a vase or
perhaps even worn as a
corsage on International
Women's Day.

Fluffy yellow, lightly scented, ball-shaped mimosa flowers cover the ends of small branches from the end of winter to early spring.

Mimosa is said to encourage a wealth of attributes, including sensitivity, advancement, success, leadership, healing and joy. It is also the recognised emblem of International Women's Day. International Women's Day or, as it is more commonly called in Italy, La Festa della Donna, is celebrated on 08 March by the giving and receiving of mimosa blossom. Women's Day originated in New York in 1909 and 8 March became a national holiday in the US after women gained suffrage in 1917. In more recent times, women now hand the flowers to other women – be it friends, sisters, mothers or other female relatives, as a sign of solidarity.

Mimosa is the perfect token with which to celebrate not only International Women's Day but also the success of women in general. It would make an ideal gift for a female friend to celebrate her promotion, or motherhood, or even just as a sign of female friendship.

Daffodils

FLOWERING PERIOD
March to April

CARE Daffodils that have just been cut ooze a sticky sap that shortens the life of other flowers around them. If you are combining daffodils with different flowers, give them an hour in water alone. Keep ends trimmed regularly and water refreshed daily and these should last for up to a week.

PRESENTATION A simple bunch of daffodils is always a welcome sight, but they also work well in both bouquets and arrangements.

TOXIC

Immortalised by William Wordsworth in one of the poems most recited by schoolchildren, the daffodil is celebrated in Wales as one of its national emblems and blooms in perfect time for St David's Day in March.

The humble daffodil is also enjoyed as a symbol of Easter and it comes into full flower just as the Christian church is celebrating the renewal of life and the resurrection. For this reason, the daffodil is also known as the Lent lily or Easter lily. In some places, and in Wales in particular, the two things come together in a tradition known as 'the flowering of the graves' on Palm Sunday. Graves are cleaned, whitewashed and weeded before being decked with garlands of daffodils and spring flowers.

The bright yellow, cheery nature of the daffodil, together with its connections to Easter, make it a perfect celebratory flower and, given its widespread availability in the spring, it's an easy to come by, simple gift.

Hyacinths

FLOWERING PERIOD
December to April

CARE Cut off the slightly bulbous ends of the stems and place in clear, fresh water. Refresh water daily and place a piece of charcoal in the water to stop the ends of the plants from becoming slimy.

PRESENTATION As well as being used as a cut flower, indoor displays of hyacinths using peat-free compost in terracotta pots with drainage holes, covered with moss, are also popular.

TOXIC

The wonderful perfume of the hyacinth heralds the start of the new year. When all around is gloomy and dark, what better than a crisp, white hyacinth to cheer up a room and fill it with scent?

The hyacinth's name can be traced back to a young Greek boy named Hyakinthos. According to Ovid's *Metamorphoses*, two gods – Apollo (the sun god) and Zephyr (the god of the west wind) – were vying for the attention of Hyakinthos. One day, while Apollo was teaching Hyakinthos how to throw a discus, Zephyr, in a jealous rage, blew the discus back, killing Hyakinthos with a blow to the head. Apollo named the flower that grew from Hyakinthos's blood in his honour. Despite the grisly story of its origin, often seen as symbolising sport or play, the blue hyacinth also represents sincerity. It has also been seen to symbolise rashness (as shown in the behaviour of Zephyr) and sorrow at an act wrongly committed.

An ideal present to celebrate Christmas or the New Year, hyacinths are the perfect gift for new beginnings. Additionally, they celebrate a fresh start in a relationship or make a good form of apology for rash behaviour.

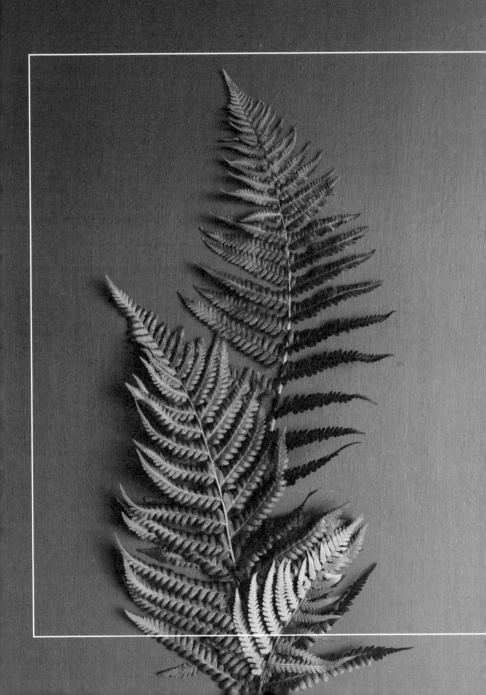

Foliage

Pine

FOR CALM

FLOWERING PERIOD
Year round

CARE If placing in a vase,
cut a 'V' shape into the end
of the pine's stem to allow
it to drink as much water as
possible. However, pine will
also last well out of water.

PRESENTATION In
addition to making a good
accompaniment to winter
flowers, such as bold
amaryllises, pine makes
excellent decorations in the
form of garlands, wreaths
and hanging branches.

Pine is a very useful type of foliage as it is
widely available and grows all year round.
Its uses are varied, but its meanings are
ones of calm and happiness.

In Japan, it was once a custom to place a
pine branch over the entrance to a house to
encourage happiness in the home. It is also
the Tree of Peace within the Native American
Iroquois Confederacy.

The scent of pine is widely used in aromatherapy
as it is fresh, soft and forest like. It is used to
lessen the symptoms of asthma and coughing,
soothe rheumatism and treat anxiety and
depression. The fragrance is also said to
increase a sense of family well-being, harmony
and goodwill, as well as releasing energy, clearing
emotional blocks and increasing intuition.
It is the perfect calming foliage.

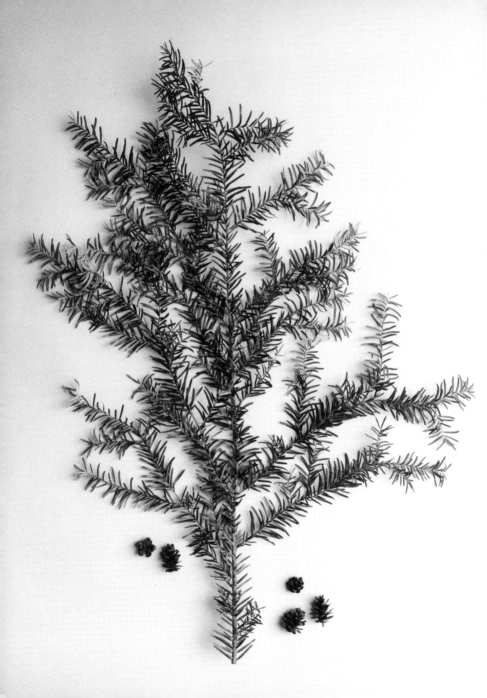

Eucalyptus

⊖ FOR CALM

⊕ FLOWERING PERIOD
Year round

⊕ CARE Eucalyptus lasts
particularly well, often for as
long as two weeks; if keeping
in a vase, trim ends regularly
and refresh water daily.

⊗ PRESENTATION
Eucalyptus is a useful
foliage for many things –
it is great in a bouquet or
arrangement and also looks
good when worked into a
wreath. It is easy to dry and
sits well alongside other
dried flowers.

*The foliage pictured here
has been dried.*

Eucalyptus is available all year and is one of
the most accessible and commonly used types
of foliage. Originally native to Australia, it is
now grown in many parts of the world, and
while there are many varieties, it is *Eucalyptus
gunnii* (circular leaves) and *Eucalyptus parvi*
(more delicate, long, thin leaves) that are
the two most frequently used.

Eucalyptus is well known for its calming and
healing properties and it is an anti-inflammatory
and decongestant. Folklores state that carrying
eucalyptus leaves encourages good health
and that hanging a piece of eucalyptus over
a sickbed will encourage healing.

Eucalyptus is a good foliage to include
when gifting flowers to help promote calm
and healing.

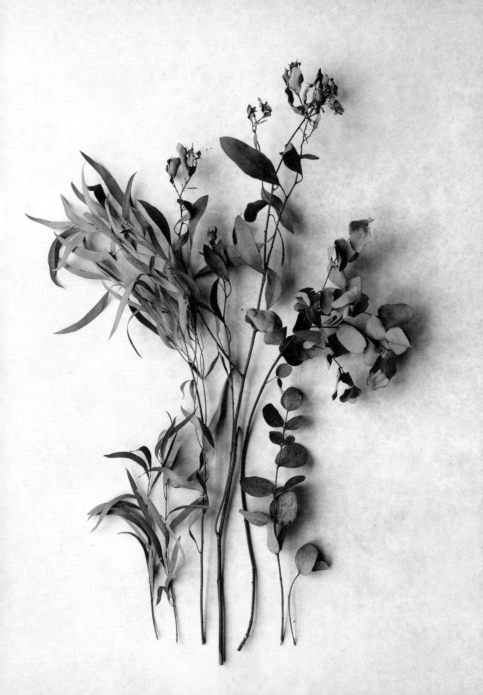

THE LANGUAGE OF

Moss

⊖ FOR CALM

✿ FLOWERING PERIOD
Year round

⊕ CARE If moss is drying out,
spritz it with a water spray
or soak it in water. Check the
moss regularly to see that it
remains moist.

⚲ PRESENTATION Often
used to cover the top of
potted plants, moss is also a
good base for floral wreaths
or other structures where
plants need a constant
water supply.

Like a plush green carpet spread across walls
and woodlands, moss can thrive in some of
the least-hospitable environments. In winter
it protects the roots of trees and plants from
freezing weather and ground frosts and provides
birds with soft material for their nests. During
warmer months, a blanket of moss on a
woodland floor provides somewhere soft to sit
and rest. Moss has been compared to a mother's
love due to its constant presence, and its warm
embrace inspires calm and reassurance.

Moss is so important to the ecosystem that it
is a protected species and you should not dig
it up yourself when out walking. Always find
a commercial outlet that sells properly and
sustainably foraged moss.

Often overlooked as a token in its own right,
added to another plant or flower, moss gives
an extra layer of meaning to a floral gift.
For example, moss is sometimes used when
potting up indoor bulbs. If using hyacinths,
which symbolise new beginnings, they could
be combined with moss to produce a gift offering
reassurance that there are good times ahead.

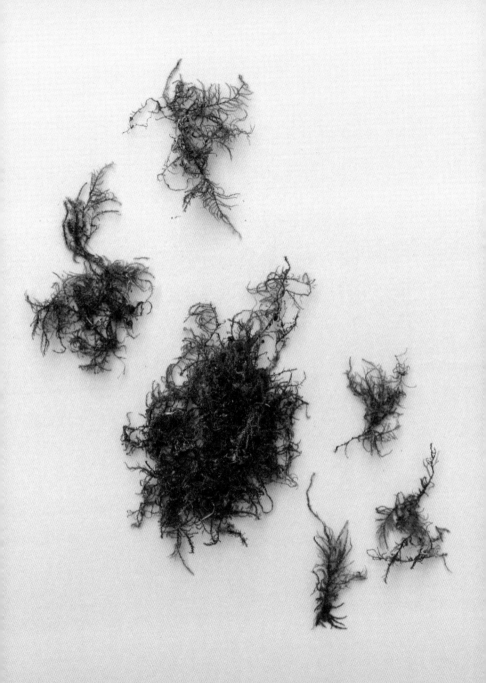

Artemisia

◎ FOR LOVE

⊛ FLOWERING PERIOD
July to September

⊕ CARE Strip back the
many bottom leaves to
ensure there are none
below the water line.
Trim ends regularly
and refresh water daily.

⚬ PRESENTATION
Artemisia is a good foliage
to use in a bouquet or
arrangement as it is light
and not too bulky. It also
dries very well and looks
good in a wreath.

⚠ TOXIC

*The foliage pictured here
has been dried.*

With its silvery leaves, reddish stems and small
yellow flowers, artemisia is a pretty foliage with
a light airiness that makes it popular with florists.
Its scientific name, *Artemisia absinthium*,
comes from *absinthus*, meaning 'without
sweetness', and the word 'absence' is also
derived from its name. As it is a bitter-tasting
herb, it is known as the emblem of separation,
absence and the torments of love, all of which
are associated with bitterness.

Artemisia dries very well and its everlasting
quality means that it is also enduring. It would
be the perfect plant to give to someone from
whom you are about to be separated, expressing
sadness at parting but also reassuring them of
the enduring nature of your love.

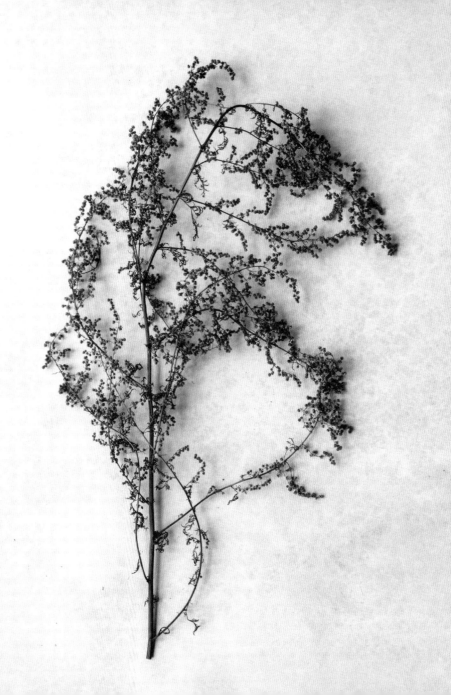

Smokebush

FOR LOVE

FLOWERING PERIOD
July to August

CARE Crush, cut or
break woody branches in
an upwards motion, leaving
a longer cut-surface area
so that more water can be
taken in. Trim ends regularly
and refresh water daily and
this foliage will last at least
a week.

PRESENTATION
These smoky plumes
add a lightness of touch
to both bouquets and
arrangements. They
also look good in dried
flower wreaths.

*The foliage pictured here
has been dried.*

Smokebush is a plant with dark red or purple foliage, but when it flowers it appears to be wreathed in smoke, hence its name. Its scientific name, *cotinus*, is derived from the Greek word *cotunos*, meaning 'wild olive tree', but it is in fact a member of the cashew family. It is even more surprising, then, that very unusual-looking, minute flowers which look like fluffy clouds cluster together to replace the dark leaves. These are the perfect texture to add to floral pieces as they are light and do not crowd other flowers.

Smokebush symbolises rare beauty, so it is the ideal foliage to incorporate when conveying a message of romantic love and/or admiration.

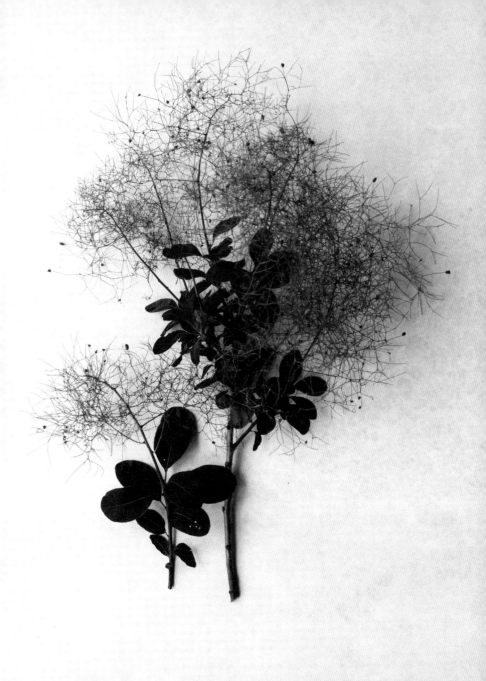

THE LANGUAGE OF

Ivy

FOR LOVE

FLOWERING PERIOD
Year round

CARE If keeping ivy in
water, trim ends regularly
and refresh water daily.

PRESENTATION Because
of its toxic nature, it is not
a good idea to have ivy in
bouquets where the leaves
can come into prolonged
contact with the holder's
skin. Ivy looks good where
it can be wrapped around
something – a structure in
a room – or trailing from
an arrangement or vase.

TOXIC

For a seemingly ubiquitous and easy-to-find
plant, ivy is one of the most symbolic, and signifies
eternal life to both Christians and pagans alike.
It is also thought to guard against negative
energies and impending dangers.

The most popular meanings of ivy are those that
are most literally associated with its behaviour.
Ivy gently wraps its foliage around old buildings
and trees, and once it has spread its tendrils
across these structures, it is not easily separated
from them. If a tree is felled, the ivy does not die
off but continues to grow around the tree on
the ground. Only killing off the ivy itself will
successfully separate it from that which it
embraces. This devotion has led to ivy being
perceived as the emblem of happy love, marriage,
friendship within wedlock and wedded love.
Its steadfast behaviour is seen to represent great
friendship and true love and is a sign of fidelity.

Ivy is a perfect plant to include in wedding
celebrations, or to incorporate in a gift for
the happy couple as they move into a new
home together.

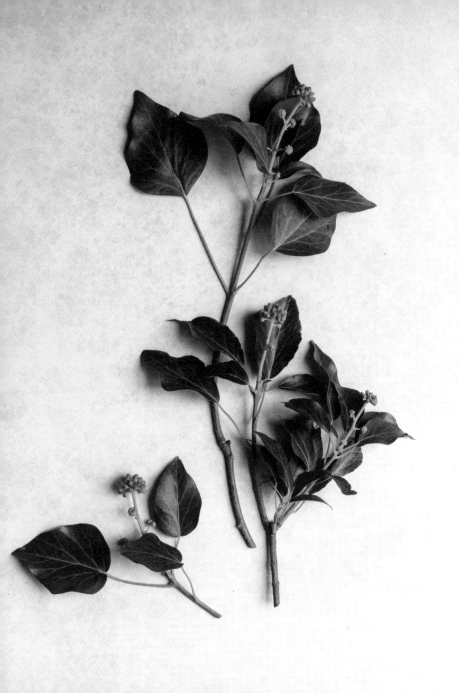

Myrtle

FOR LOVE

FLOWERING PERIOD
July to August

CARE Crush, cut or break
woody branches in an
upwards motion, leaving
a longer cut-surface area
so that more water can be
taken in. Trim ends regularly
and refresh water daily.

PRESENTATION Myrtle
works well in both bouquets
and arrangements.

TOXIC

Myrtle is an evergreen shrub with small leaves
and cream, pink-tinted flowers in the summer,
which are followed by purple-black berries,
that can be seen forming in the picture here.
Said to be sacred to Demeter, the Greek
goddess of the harvest and agriculture, and
Aphrodite, goddess of love, this glossy green
foliage is also a Hebrew symbol of marriage,
so it has come to be seen as an emblem of
chastity, fidelity, prosperity and good luck
in love and marriage.

With its aromatic leaves and heady meanings
of love and fidelity, myrtle is the perfect plant
to include in a romantic gesture – it was used in
the Duchess of Cambridge's wedding bouquet.

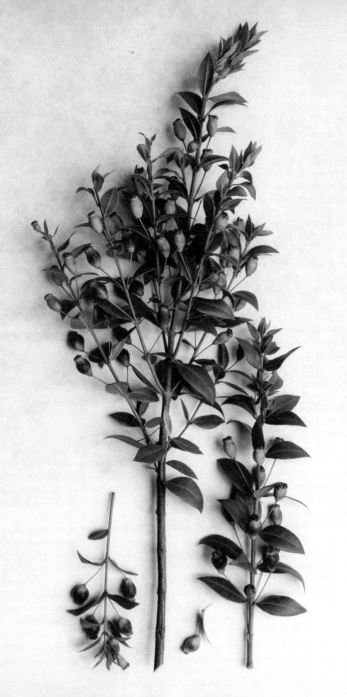

THE LANGUAGE OF

Hawthorn

△ FOR SUCCESS

⊛ FLOWERING PERIOD
April to May

⊕ CARE Crush, cut or
break woody branches in
an upwards motion, leaving
a longer cut-surface area
so that more water can
be taken in. Take care when
handling the branches of
hawthorn as they have
thorns, as their name
suggests. Trim the stems
regularly and refresh the
water daily.

 PRESENTATION
A few branches or sprigs
in a jug to bring luck into a
house is a simple gesture,
but these stems can also
be incorporated into
arrangements. They
are too thorny to include
in bouquets.

The hawthorn is known by a variety of different names, including the Beltane tree, the May blossom, the May tree, the whitethorn and the quick. In Ireland it is also known as the faerie tree, as it is said to guard the entrance to the faerie realm, and it is still considered bad luck to harm one. You may, however, collect sprigs of flowers during May to place in and around the home to banish evil spirits or misfortune.

At dawn on Beltane, 1 May, men and women would bathe in the morning dew of the hawthorn blossom to increase wealth, health, luck, good fortune and beauty. Although its pagan origins are centuries old, there modern Beltane celebrations still take place in the twenty-first century.

Nowadays, on May Day, it is the custom in Ireland to hang strips of cloth or ribbons on a hawthorn to make a wish. This is also done to ask Brigid (a goddess of pre-Christian Ireland) to bless the cloth, as these are then used in healing. Hawthorn is also one of the woods used in the hand-fastening ritual in a wedding, where the hands of a couple are wrapped together in a piece of cloth, as it will ensure a lasting relationship.

The hawthorn is also known as a tree of protection, and so it will often be found growing near a house.

THE LANGUAGE OF

Ferns

⬡ FOR SUCCESS

✿ FLOWERING PERIOD
Year round – green in spring
and summer, brown in
autumn and winter.

⊕ CARE If you are keeping
them fresh in water, trim
ends regularly and refresh
water daily. If using as a
dried plant, they can first
be flattened by placing
them between large sheets
of newspaper and placing
something heavy on them,
like a book or even a
heavy rug.

⚭ PRESENTATION Ferns
look good as background
foliage in arrangements,
or in very small quantities
in a bouquet. Dried ferns
look wonderful in dried
arrangements and wreaths,
and ferns also respond well
to being pressed.

*The foliage pictured here
has been dried.*

There are many types of fern, but it is the
Dryopteris variety, which are commonly known
as bracken, that is most often used for floral
arrangements. Some are evergreen but others
fade to a browner colour and crisper texture in
autumn and winter, and these are the most
sought after.

Ferns have their own collection of folktales
attached to them – place a frond of bracken
under a pillow in order to come up with a solution
to a perplexing problem in your sleep. To the
indigenous Maori of New Zealand ferns represent
new life and new beginnings, and to the Japanese
they symbolise family happiness and hope for
future generations. Whichever viewpoint you
look at it from, ferns are associated with
happiness and luck for the future.

You could either include ferns in an arrangement
or bouquet for a loved one or give a pressed piece
of bracken to wish them luck and happiness.

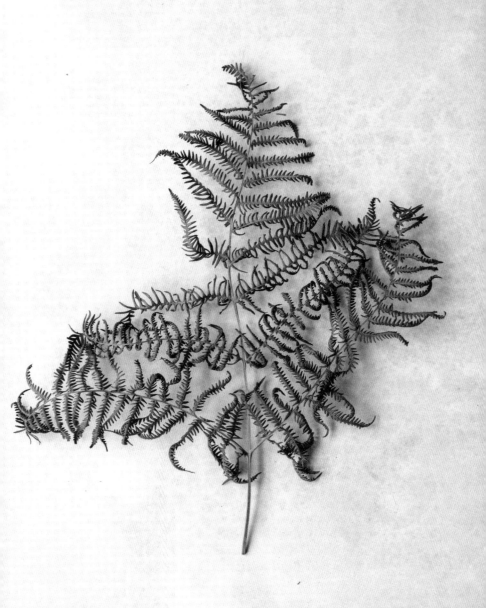

Holly

△ FOR SUCCESS

✿ FLOWERING PERIOD
November to February

⊕ CARE If you are keeping
them in water, trim stems
regularly and refresh
water daily.

♡ PRESENTATION
Holly is not suitable
to use in bouquets due
to its prickly leaves, nor
does it work particularly
well in arrangements.
Place snippets in small
glass vases scattered
around the house,
mixed with ivy for table
decorations, or use to
make a holly wreath.

⚠ TOXIC

When we see holly, we most often think of
Christmas, when we see it on greeting cards,
used to decorate houses and in people's
gardens. Holly was very important to a
Victorian Christmas, where it was used to
decorate picture frames, mantelpieces, gas
lamps and the festive table.

Holly, with it glossy, green, prickly leaves
and deep-red berries, is traditionally a symbol
of foresight, courage, good luck, good cheer,
domestic happiness and wisdom. Folklore tells
us that it became an emblem of foresight as it
has prickly leaves towards the bottom of its
bush to protect it from grazing cattle, but
higher up the plant, out of reach of animals,
the leaves lose their sharpness.

Holly was also used in divination by Victorians
– young girls would place a sprig of holly under
their pillow in the hope that they would dream
of their future husband. Its fortune-telling
powers were also tested by placing tiny candles
on the leaves and floating them in water – if the
leaves stayed afloat, then the venture in question
would succeed, if they sank, then it was best
not to go ahead with the plans.

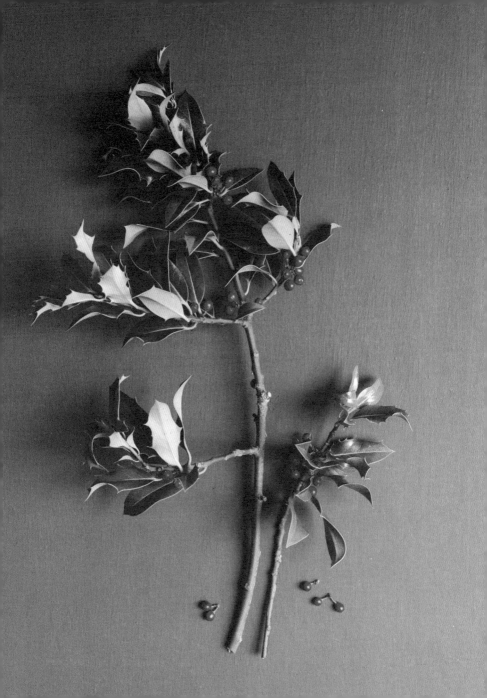

As a bringer of good fortune, holly was sometimes placed on a bedpost to encourage sweet dreams, and it was planted near homes for luck and protection. It was strongly believed to protect against misfortune.

All of these uses means that holly carries a much more complex meaning than a simple 'Merry Christmas'. It is the perfect gift to wish someone luck and success in their life – perhaps in their new home or venture.

Viburnum

⊖ FOR CALM

⊕ FLOWERING PERIOD
May to June

⊕ CARE Trim the ends
regularly and refresh
the water daily.

⊗ PRESENTATION This
floral foliage looks pretty
in both bouquets and
arrangements.

There are many types of viburnum, some snowball-shaped and others with winter flowers and berries, but it is the delicate white flowers that can be found in early summer that are prized by florists. These small white flowers add an elegant touch to bouquets and arrangements alongside the structure from the viburnum.

Viburnum has been attributed the powers of focus, meditation, relaxation and pain relief and so would make the perfect gift for someone recuperating from a period of stress or illness who needs some calm during their recovery.

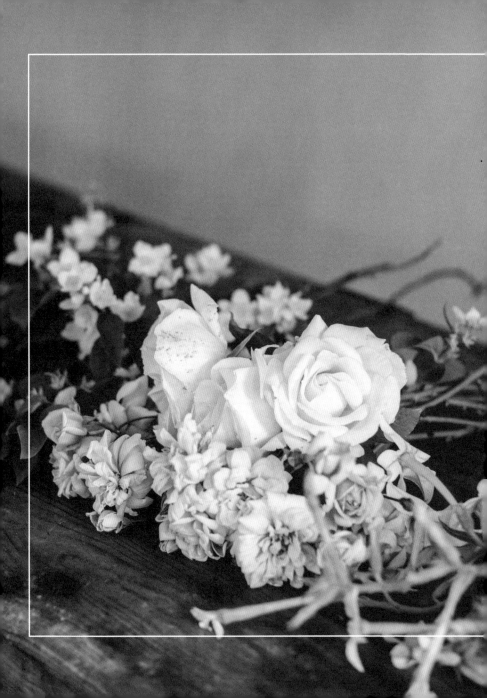

Bouquets

to

<u>Share</u>

How to make
a simple bouquet

You don't need to be a brilliant florist with a wonderful 'spiralling' technique, or have a vast selection of flowers to make a beautiful bouquet.

SELECTING YOUR FLOWERS

When choosing your flowers, you may be drawn to them because of their shape, their colour or their texture – you might want to go for big, bold blooms or make something delicate from wispy wild flowers. You might like certain colours, which can add a further layer of meaning to your bouquet. Equally, you may be attracted to particular textures – flowers come in all sorts of smooth, glossy, feathery, velvety, crinkly varieties and it is likely you will have more than one of these in your bouquet. Most of all, inspired by the previous pages, you will hopefully have selected at least one of the flowers because of its meaning.

But before this all starts to sound too complicated, it is important to note that you can create a wonderful floral piece with between three and five types of flower. Your bouquet will have the most impact if it has one of each of the three fs: foliage, focal and floaty.

FOLIAGE

This is generally a type of greenery, such as eucalyptus (see page 166) or viburnum (see page 185), which is completely or predominantly made up of leaves. A twiggy branch with small stems, like spirea (see page 018), could also fall into this category. The foliage is there to give overall shape to the bouquet and to create some space between the flowers.

FOCAL FLOWERS

These tend to be the attention-grabbing flowers such as roses (see page 075), anemones (see page 130) or ranunculus (see page 014). They are often, though not always, round in shape and heavier than the floaty flowers.

FLOATY FLOWERS

These are the more delicate flowers that soften up the harsh lines of the foliage and add some lightness between the foliage and the focal flowers. They often have flatter heads than the focal flowers.

Some flowers fit into more than one of the categories. A climbing plant like honeysuckle (see page 062) or jasmine (see page 032) is a way of adding both shape and delicate flowers to your bouquet and could be seen as both foliage and a floaty flower. The important thing is to have a mixture of the three types of form. In the list below you will therefore see some flowers that appear in more than one section.

FOLIAGE

Artemisia
Dogwood
Eucalyptus
Ferns
Hawthorn
Holly
Honeysuckle
Ivy
Jasmine
Magnolia
Mistletoe
Mock orange
Pine
Smokebush
Spirea
Viburnum

FOCAL FLOWERS

Amaryllis
Anemones
Camellias
Carnations
Chrysanthemums
Clematis
Daffodils
Dahlias
Delphiniums
Foxgloves
Gladioli
Hellebores
Hollyhocks
Hyacinths
Hydrangeas
Iris
Lilacs
Lilies
Lupins
Narcissi
Peonies
Ranunculus
Roses
Snapdragons
Stocks
Sunflowers
Tulips
Zinnias

FLOATY FLOWERS

Alstroemeria
Ammi
Aquilegia
Bleeding heart
Blossom
Campanula
Clematis
Cosmos
Cow parsley
Dogwood
Forget-me-not
Fritillary
Geraniums
Hawthorn
Hollyhocks
Honeysuckle
Japanese
  anemones
Jasmine
Magnolia
Mimosa
Mock orange
Muscari
Nasturtiums
Nicotiana
Nigella
Pansies
Phlox
Poppies
Snapdragons
Solomon's seal
Spirea
Strawflowers
Sweet peas
Verbena
Wallflowers
Zinnias

Building your bouquet

Once you have selected your flowers and foliage, lay them out in front of you so that you can easily pick them up as you hold your bouquet in your other hand. This will make your job much easier. Make sure you strip back any leaves towards the bottom of the stems and be especially careful to remove any thorns from roses, if you are using them.

Start to build your bouquet. There is no right or wrong way to go about this, but it is very important to make sure that you hold your stems gently so that they are not crushed. Begin by placing a piece of foliage flat in your hand and then add a focal flower on top of that, followed by one or two of your floaty flowers and keep building until you have the desired shape or size. Keep your hand flat and hold the flowers loosely as you add them. Continue to add flowers of different lengths to shape the bouquet.

The individual stems do not need to be straight in order to be included. Sometimes imperfect ones are best.

If there is a bend in a flower, then use it to your advantage, follow the line that it is taking, and this will help to make your bouquet look more natural.

As you build up your layers, it is a good idea to keep the lighter stems in the middle, partly to add lightness to the bouquet but also because the lighter stems are the most easily crushed. Ensure nothing is criss-crossed, you should just have flowers gently nestled on top of one another. Layer some flowers lower and others higher to build up volume. As a general rule, keep floaty flowers higher and focal ones lower and tucked in a little deeper as they are heavier, and this will result in a more even bouquet.

Rotate your bunch, while keeping it in your hand, so that you add flowers to the back and sides as well as the front to give the bouquet some 3D shape – it does not need to be a uniform shape or pattern, and nature can be quite asymmetrical, but you do need to have flowers at the back as well as the front so that your bouquet is not completely flat.

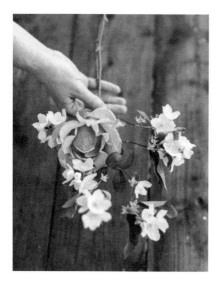

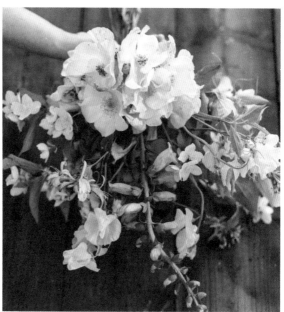

Finishing your bouquet

Once you have achieved your desired shape, to finish off the bouquet, tie a piece of string (ideally a natural one, which will biodegrade easily) around the end of the stems, about 5–8cm from the bottom, depending on the overall length of the bunch. Tie a knot and cut any loose ends. Then trim the stems to make sure they are all roughly the same length at the bottom. Finally, if you have some ribbon available, use this to cover the string and tie a bow to one side for a final flourish.

If it is a while until you are able to give the bouquet, it is a good idea to keep the stems hydrated. The easiest way to do this is to keep the flowers in a vase or jar of water until it is time to hand them over. Alternatively, it is possible to buy eco wraps, which are pieces of a material that looks a bit like a baby's nappy. They are soaked in water before being wrapped around the stems and will keep the flowers fresh for several hours. They are biodegradable and so are an environmentally friendly option. Please don't use cellophane or plastic if you can avoid it. If you do choose to keep your flowers in water, it might be better to add the ribbon later so that it doesn't get wet.

HOW TO PUT A BOUQUET TOGETHER

Here are six suggested bouquet recipes, put together at different times of year and with a range of meanings. The ingredients for each bouquet were determined by the message that I wanted to send and the flowers that were in season at that time (or, in the case of winter, the dried flowers that were in stock). Some bouquets are larger than others, so the quantity of flowers can be scaled up or down, depending on your budget and/or desired impact, whether it's a small gesture of friendship or a grand declaration of love.

In each case there is a mixture of the three Fs (see page 188 – focal, floaty and foliage), but as long as there is a combination of these, and ideally one of each type, the bouquet will take shape easily. Depending on the time of year that you're making the bouquet, you can swap one seasonal flower for another. For example, peonies are only available for a short period in May to June, so if you want to make the bouquet for a carefree romantic (see page 198) in

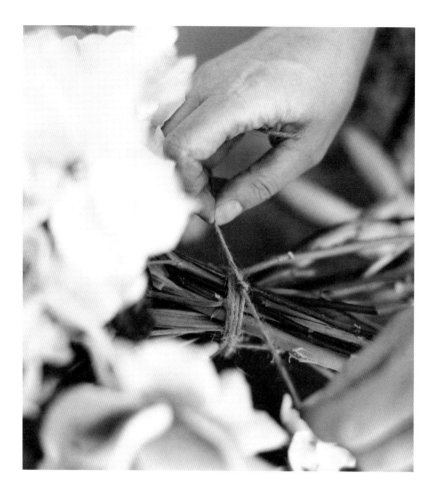

August, you could use dahlias instead, as they are also focal flowers and carry the same meaning of romantic love. Likewise, if you're making the bouquet for comfort (see page 196) in the spring rather than summer, then swap the poppies for earlier-flowering

anemones, and add some forget-me-nots in place of one of the floaty forms. Once you've checked the meanings of the flowers against their flowering period, the possibilities are endless and there is great scope for creativity.

Bouquet for new beginnings

6 × HONEYSUCKLE
for a happy home (page 062)

5 × ROSES
for love (page 075)

3 × FOXGLOVES
for success and energy
(page 106)

3 × MOCK ORANGE
for calm (page 040)

6 × SWEET PEAS
for joy (page 026)

This bouquet was made in early summer, when roses are in their first flush, bees are buzzing around the foxgloves and the honeysuckle and mock orange leave delicious scent in the garden. Sweet peas adorn trellises, and all seems happy and calm at home.

Given honeysuckle's traditional associations with a happy home, and the availability of other flowers with meanings including love, success and joy (as well as a little calm), this bouquet would be ideal for a couple starting out on a new life together in their first home.

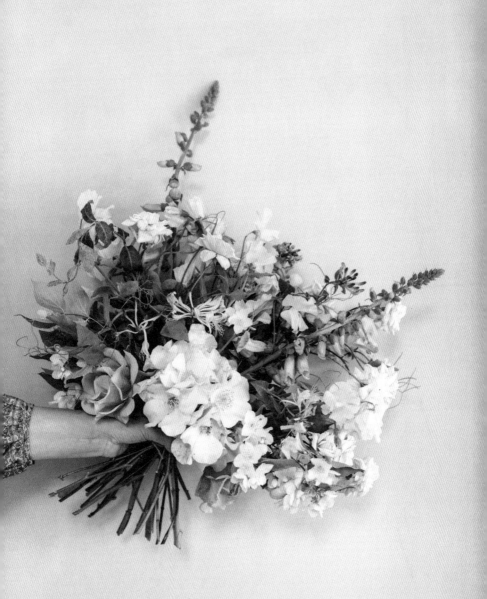

Bouquet
for comfort

9 × MARIGOLDS
for grief and consolation
(page 136)

5 × POPPIES
for grief and remembrance
(page 144)

3 × MOCK ORANGE
for calm (page 040)

5 × ROSES
for love and friendship
(page 075)

5 × CLEMATIS
for love and understanding
(page 066)

A midsummer bouquet made when the marigolds first appear. In spite of their cheerful orange and yellow tones, marigolds are traditionally associated with grief and consolation. They coincide with beautiful poppies, well known as a symbol of remembrance, and clematis, with its empathetic attributes, as well as mock orange, known for its calming effect. Roses, the ultimate symbol of love, take on a meaning of friendship rather than passionate love here.

It's hard to imagine that such a pretty combination could convey a sad message, but for this reason this bouquet should bring a smile to the recipient's face at a time when they need a little comfort.

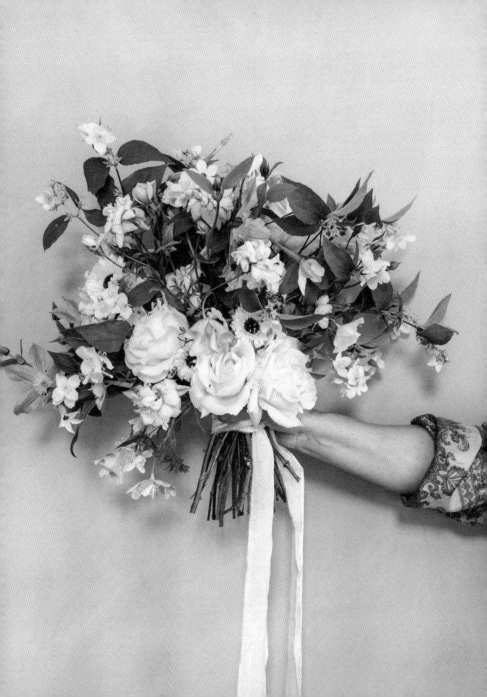

Bouquet for the carefree romantic

5 × PEONIES
for romantic love (page 122)

3 × DELPHINIUMS
for lightness and joy (page 022)

3 × MOCK ORANGE
for calm (in case you get
dizzy with love! – page 040)

5 × ROSES
for love (page 075)

5 × AMMI MAJUS
for lightness and joy (page 020)

This bouquet was made in the height of summer, when nature gives us sunshine, long evenings, and many of our favourite flowers. All of these make for a heady combination, and together are a suitable token when you're in the carefree stages of falling in love. Peonies are well-known symbols of romantic love and roses are associated with all kinds of affection. These staples are joined by joyous flowers such as delphiniums and ammi, with a smattering of calming mock orange, to ensure feet are kept in at least some kind of contact with the ground!

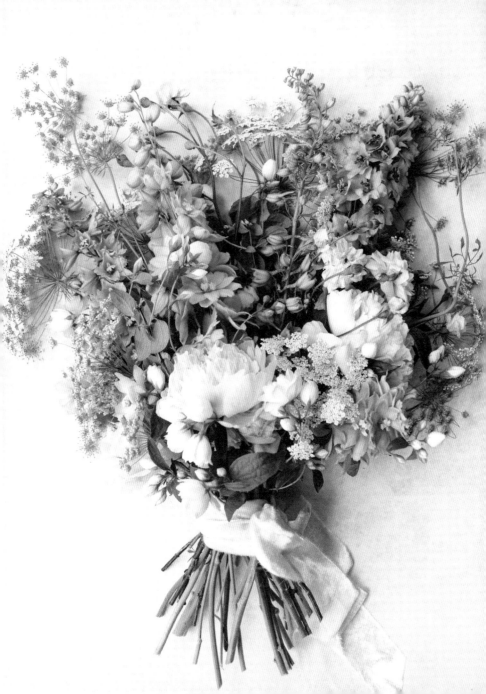

Bouquet
for new parents

6 × RANUNCULUS
for joy (page 014)

5 × SOLOMON'S SEAL
for calm and protection
(page 038)

5 × SWEET PEAS
for joy (page 026)

5 × VIBURNUM
for calm and relaxation
(page 185)

A springtime bouquet made when new life is emerging again after the long winter. The joy of fluffy ranunculus meets the very first cheerful sweet peas; Solomon's seal, associated with calm and protection, also coincides with viburnum, known for its relaxing properties. This is the ideal combination, then, to give to a parent celebrating the joyful arrival of a new member of their family, but who is perhaps also seeking a little calm. With just four types of flower, this is one of the smaller and simpler bouquets in this section.

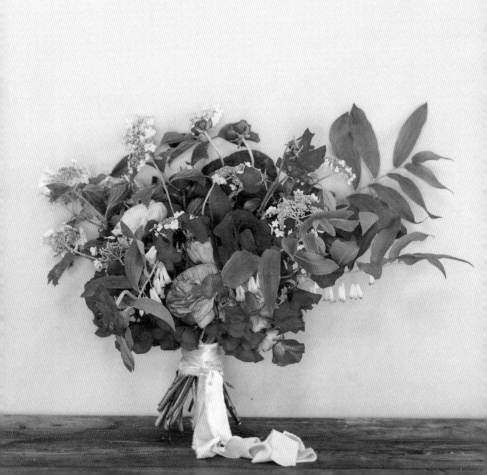

Bouquet
for passion

---

6 × CAMPANULAS
for romance (page 064)

4 × COSMOS
for joy (page 016)

8 × DAHLIAS
for love and romance (page 068)

5 × SMOKEBUSH
for romance (page 172)

A late-summer bouquet made when the dahlias have started to take over from earlier-flowering local blooms and the leaves on the smokebush are turning into smoky plumes. Campanula adds a little lightness to this bouquet and joyous cosmos adds a delicate, floaty element.

This is quite a heavy and compact bouquet, and you can use fewer dahlias and more cosmos if you want to add a lighter feel to it. This is one for maximum impact, intended as a gesture of bold and passionate love, something the showstopping dahlia is perfect for.

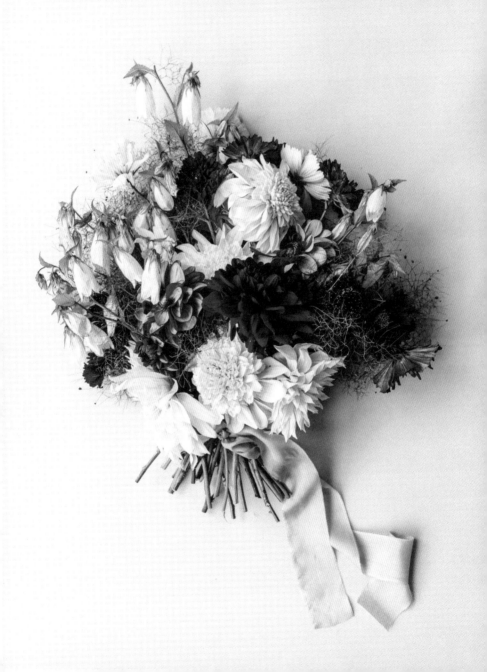

Bouquet for everlasting friendship

4 × HYDRANGEAS
for love, friendship and
community spirit (page 084)

8 × ARTEMISIA
for love (page 170)

7 × STRAWFLOWERS
for love (page 092)

6 × HELLEBORES
for steadfast friendship
(page 080)

6 × DAHLIAS
for love and friendship
(page 068)

6 × EUCALYPTUS
for calm and healing (page 168)

A bouquet that can be made at any time of year using reserves of flowers that have been dried previously (or ones bought from a grower or florist). Bear in mind that dried flowers are smaller than fresh ones since they have lost the moisture that was keeping them plump and round, so you will need more dried flowers than their fresh counterparts to make a similar impact. That said, as this particular bouquet is intended as a gesture of friendship, a smaller posy would also be appropriate, in which case the quantities listed here can be reduced.

The flowers included here are all associated with love and friendship, the scent of the dried artemisia is surprisingly strong and pleasant, even up to a year after it has been dried.

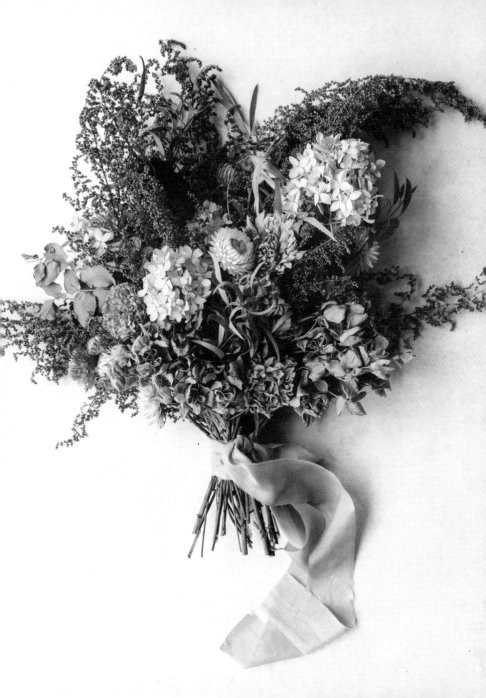

How to press flowers

Pressing flowers is a wonderful way to preserve them, and with a little patience and practice, it's not difficult. Once you have pressed your flowers, you can use them on greetings cards, as bookmarks or place settings, or even frame them. All you need are some good-quality flowers, some paper for blotting and a flower press or heavy book.

SELECTING YOUR FLOWERS

The quality of the flowers you use matters a lot when you are pressing them. The process of pressing flowers reveals a level of detail that might go unnoticed in a fresh flower, and any damage to the petals or leaves is much more obvious when it's pressed. So it's important to use flowers at their very best, either freshly picked or straight from the florist, with no nibbles on the edges, no signs of droopiness and no obvious imperfections.

Many flowers respond well to pressing, except for big blousy blooms which may retain too much moisture or have too many layers to dry out properly. With these flowers, it's still possible to press individual petals instead.

The best results come from flowers that will lie flat and retain their colour well.

FLOWERS THAT RESPOND PARTICULARLY WELL TO PRESSING ARE:

Bluebells
Cosmos
Daisies
Forget-me-nots
Geraniums
Miniature roses
Nicotiana
Nigella
Pansies
Poppies
Snowdrops

PREPARING YOUR FLOWERS

Once you have decided upon your flowers, you can choose whether you want to use the whole flower, including the stem, just the head, the petal, and so on. Prepare your flower by removing any unwanted stems or petals and ensuring that the flower is free from dirt. If necessary, dry leaves and petals with a tea towel or even some kitchen paper to ensure that they are completely dry before placing them on paper.

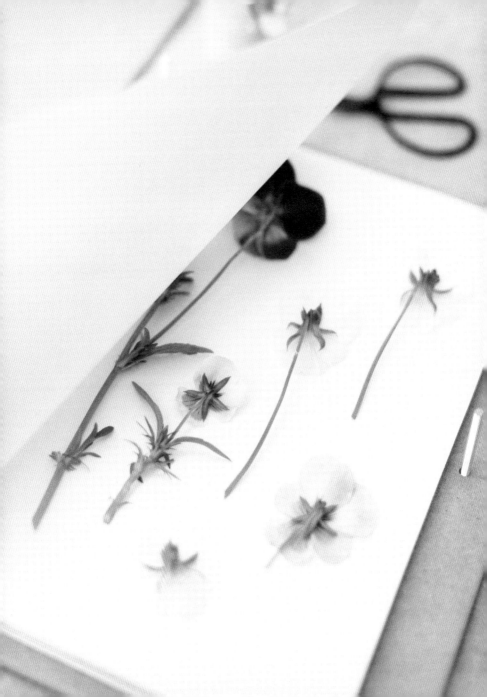

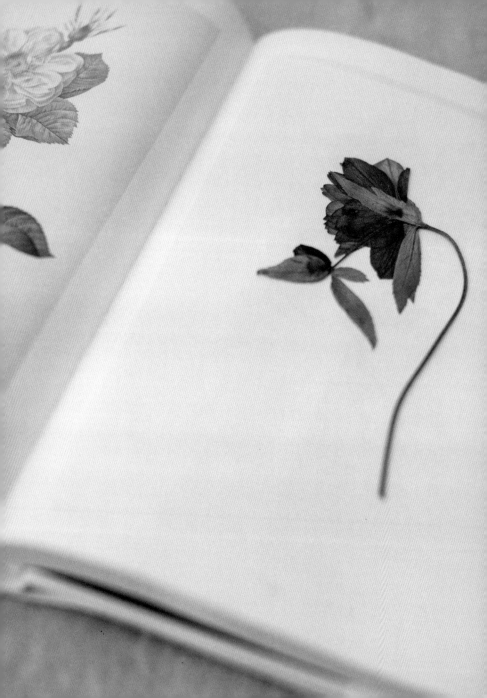

Using a flower press

Lay out the flowers you want to use in front of you. Begin with a cardboard divider on the bottom and place a fresh piece of blotting paper on top. It doesn't have to be blotting paper – printer paper, flat cardboard or plain facial tissues all work too. Avoid using kitchen paper, though, as it may leave a textured imprint on the flowers and leaves. Place your first flower on the blotting paper; if space allows, you can press more than one flower on each sheet. Having carefully positioned your flowers, lay another sheet of blotting paper carefully on top of them, then add another piece of cardboard divider on top of that. If you want to add more layers of flowers, repeat this process again, adding blotting paper on top of the divider and then the flowers and so on, almost as if you are making a lasagne.

When you have finished building your layers and are happy that everything is in position, add the wooden layer of the flower press on top of the cardboard divider and tighten the bolts to sufficiently flatten the flowers, but not so much that they are squashed and become damaged.

If you don't have a flower press, a big, heavy book works just as well. If it is not a valuable book, and you don't mind a few marks being left behind, then you can simply place the flowers carefully between the pages. If you wish to protect the book, then place blotting paper on either side of the flowers and use the pages as if they were the cardboard dividers. Make sure you leave a good number of pages between each flower/set of flowers to avoid any lumps showing, as book pages are much thinner than cardboard.

Place the flower press or book somewhere warm and dry to encourage the flowers to dry out, but not too hot so as to ruin them completely. Leave for 1–2 weeks before either unscrewing the press or gently opening up the book and removing the flowers. This is a very delicate stage as the flowers can sometimes stick to the pages. If you need to, you can use tweezers to gently lift the flowers rather than forcing them with your fingers and tearing them.

Once you have your pressed flowers, you can either use them immediately or store them carefully at room temperature in tissue paper until you want to use them.

How to dry flowers

Dried flowers are a little bit like fermented foods, in that it is wonderful to have a reserve of blooms to use when the flowers we love are no longer in season. They are perfect to see us through the winter months when we don't want to fly flowers in from overseas.

The process of drying flowers is fun, but results can be inconsistent and there is always some element of the experimental about it, no matter how much you practise. The following rules, however, should help you to achieve the best possible results.

It is best to dry your flowers as soon as is practical after picking or buying them. This ensures that they are in the best possible condition when the drying process begins. Make sure that anything to be dried is free from moisture, as this can encourage mould to grow, causing leaves to get slimy and preventing the actual process of drying.

Having ensured that your blooms are in the best possible condition and free from moisture, there are a few methods

that you can try but these two are the easiest and often yield the best results.

Hanging flowers to dry, upside down – Having prepared your flowers as above, strip all unwanted foliage from the stems. Gather together a small group of the flowers you want to dry, tie a length of string around them a few times, and secure with a knot, leaving enough string around the flowers to hang them up with. It is worth noting that the stems will shrink as they dry, so tie the knot tightly enough to allow for this, but not so tightly that it crushes the stems.

Leaving to dry in the vase – Perhaps the easiest method of all and this way you can also enjoy the fresh flowers as they dry. After stripping the leaves from the stems, place the blooms you wish to dry in a vase and add about 5cm of water. Then just wait – there is no need to top up the water. This works well for spray roses, hydrangeas and mimosa.

It is important that the flowers are left to dry in the correct conditions. Look for a place that is a normal room

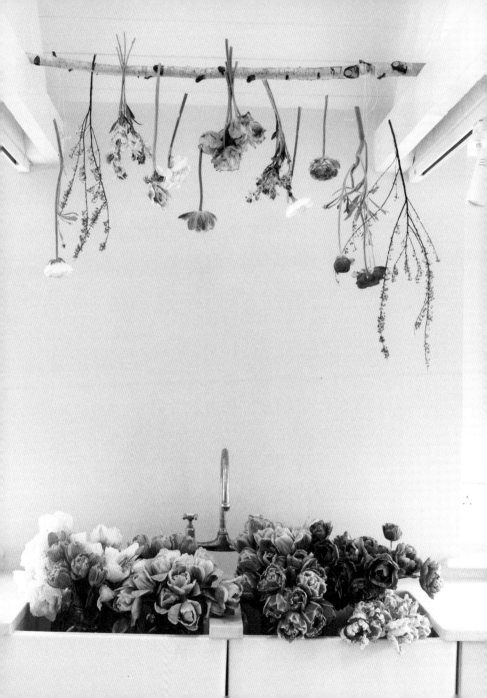

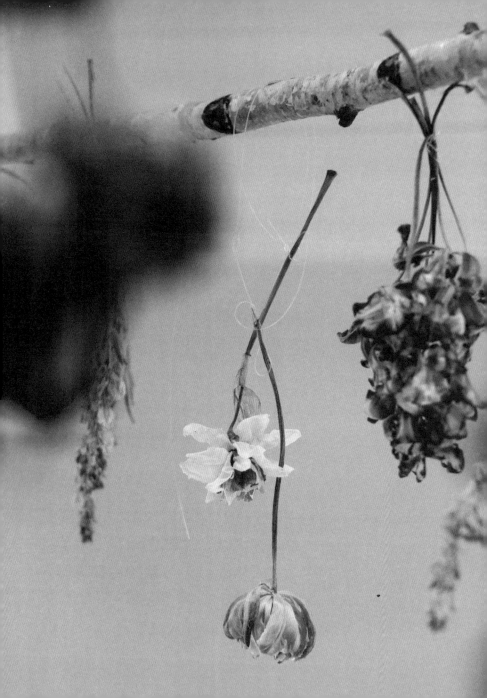

temperature – not too warm or the flowers will dry out too quickly and become brittle, out of direct sunlight and free from moisture in the air. Ideal places are an airing cupboard or a cupboard under the stairs, but as long as the space meets these three main requirements, you should yield good results. For the photography in this book, the pole that we have attached our flowers to was in the open in the studio so that the method can be easily seen, and this set up in a dark corner of a room could also work well if you don't have a cupboard.

STORAGE

Once your flowers have dried out fully, which should take about 3–5 weeks, store them in boxes lined with tissue paper or similar to ensure they do not come into contact with moisture and to keep them safe from breakages.

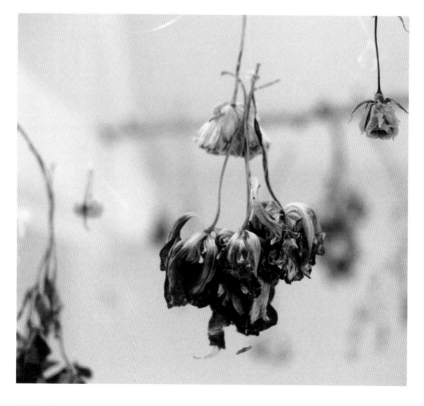

How to source flowers responsibly

AT THE FLOWER MARKET

If you're visiting a flower market for the first time, it's easy be overwhelmed by the huge variety of flowers on offer. Many of these will have been imported from overseas, however, be it from Holland, one of the largest flower-growing countries, or from further afield like South America or Africa. Ask the stallholder which, if any of their flowers, have been grown locally. Many stalls will carry a line of local flowers, too, particularly during the summer months, due to the increasing demand from florists, so it is always worth checking.

FLORISTS

As is the case with flower markets, many florists sell flowers that have been imported from overseas, particularly during the winter. Increasingly, though, they buy flowers from local growers, too, and should be able to identify these for you. These are the ones you really want and are often easily identifiable on account of their more natural, whimsical appearance.

SUPERMARKETS

If you can't get to a flower market or florist, then it is still possible to find some treasure here. Traditionally, flowers in supermarkets have been flown in from abroad and sit on the shelves wrapped in lots of plastic. More recently, the tide has been turning and some major supermarkets have now pledged to only supply flowers wrapped in paper, which is a major step forward. They are also getting better at sourcing locally grown flowers. If you are buying flowers from a supermarket, the country of origin should be clearly marked on the label, as with food, so you can ensure you are not buying flowers flown in from overseas.

FORAGING

Foraging is a wonderful way to find little snippets and gestural pieces to add to your bouquet, as well as interesting foliage. However, you need to observe some basic rules in order to forage with politeness. If you are on private land, ask permission first. Respect that some areas are off limits: public parks, front gardens and window boxes, for example, are definitely not to be touched. Make sure that you use snips so that you do not damage the rest of the plant (no ripping or pulling) and take only what you really need. When you leave with your stash, it should look as though no one has been there at all. These resources are shared by others who appreciate their beauty, and furthermore, much of nature provides a home to, and food for, insects and wildlife.

Most importantly, always make sure that you know what you are bringing back into your home. Some flowers, such as bluebells, are protected by law, and others could be toxic to pets or small children.

A NOTE ON FLORAL FOAM

All the bouquets in this book are intended to sit in a vase or vessel of water. Both florists and the public at large are becoming increasingly aware of the adverse effects of floral foam on the environment and there has been a strong movement against its use. The Royal Horticultural Society has banned its use at their flower shows, and many florists are now proudly foam free.

Although it is green in colour, its credentials are anything but – one block of floral foam contains as much plastic as at least ten plastic shopping bags, as well as formaldehyde and phenolic foam, both of which are toxic. It is not biodegradable, cannot be recycled and when it ends up in landfill, it ultimately breaks down into increasingly small microplastics, which then contaminate the food chain. It also gets into our water supply systems, leaching chemicals into the water, and the smaller particles are ingested by aquatic animals.

Further information can be found at www.sustainablefloristry.org @sustainablefloristrynetwork and @nofloralfoam

A NOTE ON CELLOPHANE

Just as we should say no to floral foam, we should also look to avoid cellophane wrapping, which is often used both to wrap bouquets and/or to create a 'pool' of water to keep the flowers hydrated while they are in transit. Cellophane, like other plastics, is not biodegradable and adds to the carbon footprint of your bouquet. Look for bouquets that are wrapped in paper or, if wrapping your own, brown recycled paper is the ideal. If you need to keep the flowers fresh en route to your recipient, either keep them in a jar of water or use a biodegradable 'nappy' which is soaked in water before being wrapped around the bottom of the flower stems. A compostable bag is secured on top.

Further information can be found at www.ecofreshbouquet.com @ecofreshbouquet

Find a grower near you

The best way to ensure provenance is to buy from a local grower, and in doing so you are directly supporting a local business.

Many flower growers belong to a national network and will have a website that will help you to locate them. Some suggestions are listed below.

FOR UK GROWERS

FLOWERS FROM THE FARM
www.flowersfromthefarm.co.uk
@flowersfromthefarm

THE BRITISH FLOWER
COLLECTIVE
www.thebritishflowercollective.com
@thebritishflowercollective

FOR US AND CANADA
GROWERS

SLOW FLOWERS
www.slowflowers.com
@myslowflowers

FOR AU GROWERS

THE GOOD BUNCH
MELBOURNE
www.thegoodbunchmelbourne.com.au
@goodbunchmelb

FOR WORLDWIDE GROWERS

FLORET
www.floretflowers.com/directory
@floretflower

Resources and Stockists

The flowers featured in this book
were grown by:

GREEN AND GORGEOUS
www.greenandgorgeousflowers.co.uk
@gandgorgeousflowers

NETTLEWOOD FLOWERS
www.nettlewoodflowers.co.uk
@nettlewoodflowers

THE LAND GARDENERS
www.thelandgardeners.com
@thelandgardeners

DAISY WORKS
www.daisyworks.co.uk
@daisyworksuk

AESME FLOWERS
www.aesme.co.uk
@aesmestudio

JUST DAHLIAS
www.justdahlias.co.uk
@justdahlias

THE REAL FLOWER COMPANY
www.realflowers.co.uk
@therealflowerco

TANGLE AND THYME
www.tangleandthyme.co.uk
@tangleandthyme

WOLVES LANE FLOWER COMPANY
www.wolveslaneflowercompany.com
@wolveslaneflowercompan

BABYLON FLOWERS
www.babylonflowers.co.uk
@babylon_flowers

DAYLESFORD FARM
www.daylesford.com
@daylesfordfarm

Resources and Stockists

Ribbons were naturally dyed by:

Vessels purchased from:

THE NATURAL DYEWORKS
(UK)
www.naturaldyeworks.com
@thenaturaldyeworks

NETTLE AND SILK
(US AND UK)
www.nettleandsilk.com
@nettle_and_silk

GOOSE VINTAGE HOME
@goose_vintage_home

NOE KUREMOTO CERAMICS
www.noekuremoto.com
@noe_kuremoto_ceramics

PETERSHAM NURSERIES
www.petershamnurseries.com
@petershamnurseries

DAYLESFORD FARM
www.daylesford.com
@daylesfordfarm

ILLYRIA POTTERY
www.illyriapottery.co.uk
@illyriapottery

Further reading

Benzakein, Erin, *Floret Farm's: A Year in Flowers* (Chronicle Books, 2020)

Brown, Claire, *The British Flowers Book* (Compass Publishing, 2018)

Connolly, Shane, *Discovering the Meaning of Flowers: Love Found, Love Lost, Love Restored* (Clearview, 2017)

Day, Anna and Jauncey, Ellie, *The Flower Appreciation Society: An A to Z of All Things Floral* (Sphere, 2015)

Dietz, S. Theresa, *The Complete Language of Flowers: A Definitive and Illustrated History* (Wellfleet Press, 2020)

Diligent, Sarah and Mazuch, William, *A Guide to Floral Mechanics* (Diligent & Mazuch, 2020)

Dumont, Henrietta, *The Language of Flowers: The Floral Offering* (BiblioLife, 2019)

Elworthy, Bridget and Courtauld, Henrietta, *The Land Gardeners: Cut Flowers* (Thames & Hudson, 2019)

Geall, Christin, *Cultivated: The Elements of Floral Style* (Princeton Architectural Press, 2020)

Hoffmann, David, *The Complete Illustrated Holistic Herbal: A Safe and Practical Guide to Making and Using Herbal Remedies* (Element, 1999)

Keville, Kathi and Green, Mindy, *Aromatherapy: A Complete Guide to the Healing Art* (Crossing Press, US, 2009)

Kirkby, Mandy, *The Language of Flowers: A Miscellany* (Arcadia Editions, 2011)

McHarg, Fleur, *The Flower Expert: Ideas and inspiration for a life with flowers* (Thames & Hudson, 2018)

Merrick, Amy, *On Flowers: Lessons from an Accidental Florist* (Artisan, 2019)

Ngo, Ngoc Minh, *Bringing Nature Home: Floral Arrangements Inspired by Nature* (Rizzoli International Publications, 2012)

Nolan, Clare, *In Bloom: Growing, harvesting and arranging flowers all year round* (Kyle Books, 2019)

Partridge, Bex, *Everlastings: How to grow, harvest and create with dried flowers* (Hardie Grant, 2020)

Potter, Anna, *The Flower Fix: Modern arrangements for a daily dose of nature* (White Lion Publishing, 2019)

Stewart, Amy, *Gilding the Lily: Inside the Cut Flower Industry* (Granta Books, 2009)

Index

Index

About

CLAIRE BOWEN

With a background in art history and, later on, environmental campaigning, Claire Bowen is a floral stylist based in South Oxfordshire. As well as creating flowers for events, she has collaborated with brands including Daylesford, Miller Harris, People Tree and Berry Bros. & Rudd.

She teaches her foam-free, abundant techniques to both newcomers and established florists from her studio in South Oxfordshire.

This is her first book.

Visit www.honeysuckleandhilda.com or follow @honeysuckle_and_hilda on Instagram

ÉVA NÉMETH

Éva Németh's love of flowers and gardens started with her childhood spent in her grandmother's garden in Hungary. Now based in Oxfordshire, Evá regularly travels all over the UK and Europe photographing beautiful gardens, and her work has featured in magazines such as *House & Garden*, *Gardens Illustrated* and *The English Garden*.

Éva also teaches photography to people from all over the world, either online or on location. Her style is best described as 'quiet observation'.

Visit www.evanemeth.com or follow @eva_nemeth on Instagram

Thanks

FROM CLAIRE

Claire would like to thank all the growers who work so hard to grow such beautiful flowers, and in particular Rachel and Ash at Green & Gorgeous and also Bridget and Henrietta at The Land Gardeners, without both of whom it would not have been possible to write this book during lockdown. Thank you to Bex Partridge for her inspiration with flower drying.

Thank you to Samantha Crisp at Ebury Press for asking me to write this book in the first place, and for all her words of encouragement and support. Thanks to Vicky Orchard for her wonderfully astute editing skills and to Éva Németh, whose beautiful photos bring this book to life. Most of all, thank you to Charles for all his love, patience and support and for holding the fort while all of this was happening.

FROM ÉVA

Thank you to all the flower growers, whether you grow flowers in a few pots outside your front door or in your garden, you are all doing such a wonderful job and you are my inspiration.

Thank you to Sam for your vision, support and your guidance. Claire, thank you for the memories from this amazing journey during these most unbelievable times.

I would also like to thank my grandmother for showing me what loving and respecting flowers and gardens really means and all the rewarding hard work involved.

1

Published in 2021 by
Ebury Press an imprint of
Ebury Publishing,
20 Vauxhall Bridge Road,
London SW1V 2SA

Ebury Press is part of the
Penguin Random House
group of companies whose
addresses can be found at
global.penguinrandom
house.com

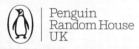

Penguin
Random House
UK

MIX
Paper from
responsible sources
FSC
www.fsc.org   FSC® C018179

DESIGN BY Imagist 2021

FIRST PUBLISHED BY Ebury Press in 2021

www.penguin.co.uk

A CIP catalogue record for this book is
available from the British Library

ISBN 9781529108132

PRINTED AND BOUND IN
China by C&C Offset Printing Co., Ltd

The authorised representative in the EEA is Penguin
Random House Ireland, Morrison Chambers, 32
Nassau Street, Dublin D02 YH68.

Penguin Random House is committed to a
sustainable future for our business, our readers
and our planet. This book is made from Forest
Stewardship Council® certified paper.

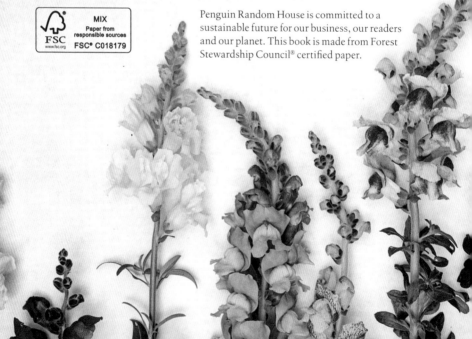